HAIRDRESSING:
TECHNICAL CERTIFICATE

ACKNOWLEDGEMENTS

The authors would like to thank Sussex Training group for the use of the premises for the photo shoot, and the students that took part in the photo shoot, especially Lauren and Oliver, for their effort and work. Thanks also to the Vocational team at Heinemann, for this great opportunity and for all the guidance and support that has been offered throughout.

Kelly Newell would like to thank her family especially her son Oliver, for their patience and support whilst writing the book.

Brenda Leonard would like to dedicate the book to Joanne and Kevin.

The authors and publisher would like to thank the following for permission to reproduce photographs:

Alamy – pages 18 (top left), 18 (top right), 18 (bottom right); Gareth Boden/Harcourt Education Ltd – page 23; CMSP (www.cmsp.com) – page 94; CORBIS – page 18 (bottom left); Goldwell – pages 141, 145; Harcourt Education/Gareth Boden – pages 15, 104, 105, 142, 160, 164, 165, 169; Harcourt Education Ltd/Gareth Boden – pages 12, 20, 84, 87 (bottom right), 88, 110, 111, 122, 124, 125, 126, 150, 151, 163, 166, 167; Harcourt Education Ltd/Chris Honeywell – pages 12, 28, 82, 86, 87 (top), 111, 127, 168; Science Photo Library – pages 93, 94, 95, 121 (top); Scissors – pages 21, 67; Wellcome Trust – page 95 (top)

HAIRDRESSING:
TECHNICAL CERTIFICATE

Kelly Newell

Brenda Leonard

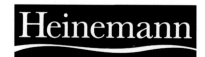

Heinemann Educational Publishers
Halley Court, Jordan Hill, Oxford OX2 8EJ
Part of Harcourt Education

Heinemann is the registered trademark of
Harcourt Education Limited

First published 2005

10 09 08 07 06 05
10 9 8 7 6 5 4 3 2 1

British Library Cataloguing in Publication Data is available
from the British Library on request.

ISBN 0 435 46177 X

Typeset and illustrated by Saxon Graphics Ltd, Derby

Original illustrations © Harcourt Education Limited, 2005

Cover design by Wooden Ark Studio
Printed by Scotprint
Cover photo: © Getty images

Acknowledgements
Every effort has been made to contact copyright holders of material reproduced
in this book. Any omissions will be rectified in subsequent printings if notice is
given to the publishers.

Websites
Please note that the examples of websites suggested in this book were up to date
at the time of writing. It is essential for tutors to preview each site before using
it to ensure that the URL is still accurate and the content is appropriate. We
suggest that tutors bookmark useful sites and consider enabling students to
access them through the school or college intranet.

CONTENTS

INTRODUCTION

This book is aimed at learners who are already working within the hairdressing industry and who require a qualification that gives them good grounding over a wide spectrum of technical subjects. It is ideal for those intending to update existing skills. The similarity of its technical elements to some of those that form part of the level 3 means that you can work towards Technical Certificate units as part of the Advanced Apprenticeship or as a stand-alone qualification.

If you are working towards the Advanced Apprenticeship framework you are required to complete your NVQ Level 3, Technical Certificate units, Key Skills and Employment Rights and Responsibilities. These four components will complete the full qualification, or you may decide to complete the Technical Certificate units alone with the option of adding the remaining components at a later date.

This book is designed to give clear advice on areas where there are opportunities to combine the components, as well as comprehensive knowledge on gaining the Technical Certificate unit requirements and meeting expectations.

You will see key skills activities throughout the book and these pieces of work will serve two purposes. Firstly, they provide evidence and extra practice for the hairdressing certificate, and secondly, they provide evidence for the key skills qualification. The key skills qualification should not involve a lot of extra work; the best key skills evidence occurs naturally. You will find lots of 'Quick tips' and 'Consider this' boxes, to act as signposts and reminders as you go through the course, and each section is completed by a 'Dear Kelly' page, in which you might find the answers to those questions you never dared to ask!

There are exercises, group activities and tasks for you to do. These are designed to help consolidate your new skills, and to allow you to share ideas with colleagues.

You will find that clear explanations are accompanied by illustrations and photographs. Who was it who said that 'a picture is worth a thousand words'? It's much easier to understand a new technique if there are pictures to refer to, to reassure you that you are getting it right.

This qualification will involve a lot of hard work and dedication on your part, but by the end of it you will be a more experienced, more competent and more confident hairdresser.

As a hairdresser, you will never stop learning. New techniques, new products and new ideas are arriving all the time, and a good hairdresser is always open to new ideas. So, take every opportunity to learn and improve your skills and gain invaluable experience along the way.

Good luck!

Brenda Leonard and Kelly Newell

SECTION 1

WORKPLACE SKILLS

UNIT 1

CONSULT WITH AND ADVISE CLIENTS

Introduction

This unit consists of one practical assignment, one written assignment and one written paper.

The practical assignment for this unit consists of two tasks. You are to provide consultation services to the client and to recommend after-care procedures and additional salon services.

The written assignment will require you to have sufficient knowledge of how to consult and advise clients with varying requirements. You will need to identify any factors that may limit the use of products or affect the provision of services. You must feel confident to give the correct advice, at the same time ensuring that you maintain goodwill and confidentiality.

The framework you are working towards will determine whether the written paper is to be marked externally or internally.

To meet the criteria, you will use the skills that you have developed during your Level 2 work, specifically in unit numbers 201 (old standards) or G9 (new standards).

To complete the practical assignment correctly, you need to ensure that you are aware of the criteria against which you will be assessed. You must also make sure that you have the correct equipment available within the salon to complete the tasks and that you are confident with the range of products available for recommendation.

Provide consultation services to the client

Good preparation is the key to success in so many areas of life – both at work and at home. For example, have you ever decorated a room? If you have, you will know that the most important part is the preparation. Washing the walls and paintwork, rubbing down the surfaces to be painted, ensuring that you use the right paint, and protecting the furniture and carpets with dust sheets are all essential. Any professional decorator will tell you that if you skimp on your preparation, it will show in the end result.

As a professional hairdresser, you should also be aware that if you skimp on your preparation the end result will be disappointing to you and the client.

Consider this

What preparations do you need to make before you start work on your client's hair?

Discuss this with the rest of your group, and draw up a list together. Then compare it with my list below. Have you covered everything? Have you thought of anything else?

- Welcome the client to the salon.
- Ensure that your client is seated comfortably.
- Consult with the client, referring to her record card in the case of an existing client, and preparing a new card in the case of a new client.
- Agree a style with the client.
- Agree any treatments and ensure that appropriate tests are carried out. As part of this, you may need to recommend special treatments to deal with hair or scalp problems. (We will be looking at this in more detail in Unit 2.)
- Ensure that the client is gowned appropriately.

Let's look at this list in more detail.

The welcome

Welcoming the client is very important. Your salon may employ a receptionist whose job it is to greet clients, or it may be part of your job. In either case, the welcome that your client receives will be her first impression of your salon.

Always provide a warm welcome to your clients

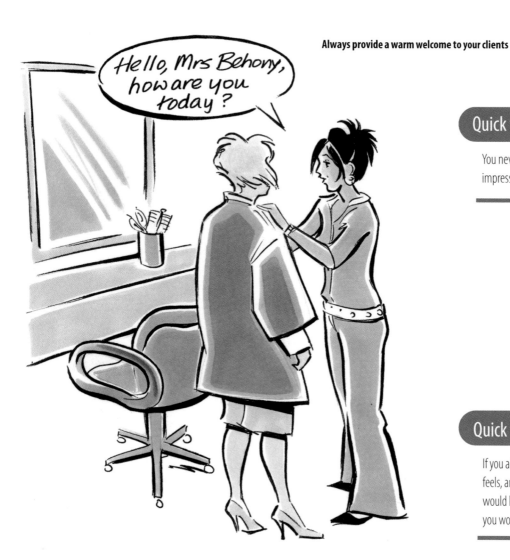

Quick tip

You never get a second chance to make a first impression!

Quick tip

If you always try to imagine how the client feels, and then treat her in the way that you would like to be treated in the same situation, you won't go far wrong.

Consider this

Try to think how you would feel if you walked into a salon and were ignored. Has it ever happened to you? Discuss this with your group, and then think about how you would like to be greeted.

"It has happened to me, and I remember exactly how I felt. There did not seem to be anywhere to hang coats, so I perched on the edge of a chair with my coat still on, feeling very uncomfortable. Everybody carried on with what they were doing, and I did not know if anybody had noticed that I had arrived. As the time for my appointment passed, I started to worry that I had been forgotten. By the time somebody finally took notice of me, I was feeling very resentful, and the stylist had to work very hard to make up for the poor welcome.

"Although I was pleased with the finished result, I never went back to that salon!"

Jasmine Pink from Crawley

Even if your salon employs a receptionist, there may be times when you have to welcome clients yourself. For example, if the receptionist is away from the desk for a moment, you should at least greet clients with a smile, ask them to take a seat, and reassure them that the receptionist will be back in a moment.

The consultation

Ensure that the client is seated comfortably

If possible, it is best to take your client into the salon, away from the reception area, when carrying out the consultation. The reception area is likely to be busy, with clients coming and going and telephones ringing, and the client will probably find it difficult to relax and concentrate on the consultation in this atmosphere.

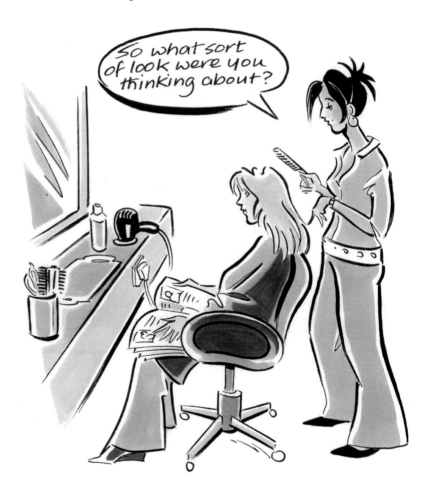

It may be helpful to seat your client in front of a mirror for the consultation

Use the client's record card

If you are meeting a new client for the first time, you will need to prepare a record card during the consultation. The first consultation is likely to take longer than future consultations, and you should not try to rush it. If you are dealing with an existing client, you should have the record card available during the consultation.

Asking questions

Your client may not know what she wants, and it is up to you to ask appropriate questions, so that you are both sure what is wanted.

Asking questions sounds quite straightforward, but you must give some thought to the sort of questions you need to ask to get the information you need. Closed questions and open questions can give you very different answers!

Closed questions: these can often be answered with a single word, and do not encourage conversation.

Open questions: these need a more detailed answer, and will help to ensure that you are certain about your client's requirements. In addition, open questions encourage conversation, and this is likely to help your client to relax.

Consider this

Look at the list of closed questions below. Can you think of an open question that could have been asked in each case? My suggestions follow, but you may find some others.

1 Is it raining outside?

2 Do you live locally?

3 Have you been on holiday this year?

4 Did you see our advertisement in the local paper?

5 Where do you work?

6 Who cut your hair last time?

Suitable open questions to ask instead could be:

1   What is the weather like outside?
2   How long did it take you to get here today?
3   What are your holiday plans for this year?
4   How did you find out about us?
5   What sort of work do you do?
6   Have you been to our salon before?

Listen to the answers

Listen with your eyes as well as your ears!

Quick tip

Beware of asking the last question in the closed list! It can seem like criticism, and apart from the fact that your client may be insulted, it is unprofessional to criticise another stylist's work.

Asking questions is a useful skill, but you also need to listen to the answers. Make careful notes of what your client tells you. When you make any suggestions, watch your client's reaction. It could be that she is saying one thing, but her body language is telling you something else.

See page 28 to learn more about body language.

The consultation checklist

During the consultation procedure, you will find it helpful to use the consultation sheet provided on pages 198–199, to ensure that you collect all the information you need. You will then have to analyse the information in order to reach a compromise between the client's requirements and what is achievable, given the facts that you have obtained.

The checklist should help you to obtain the following information.

1 Client's face shape
2 Contraindications
3 Scalp condition
4 Hair texture, hair volume (density), type, length and condition
5 Hair movement and growth patterns
6 Client's lifestyle

Let's look at each of these factors in detail.

Face shape
The shape of the face is the starting point when choosing a new hairstyle, in order to flatter some features and disguise others.

With some people, their face shape is obvious. A very long or a very round face might be hard to disguise. However, you will need to become expert at determining face shapes even when it is not easily apparent.

Try carrying out the key skills activity below on yourself (or a friend). It is probably not a good idea to try it on a client! Follow the instructions to provide evidence for key skills N2.1, N2.2 and N2.3. Carry out this activity on a number of your friends. Write down the calculations you carry out to work out what shape face each friend has. Then think of a suitable way of presenting your findings. Perhaps you could draw a pie chart and bar chart to illustrate the occurrence of each shape.

This activity alone will not provide all the evidence needed, but it will contribute to your key skills portfolio. The same activity will provide evidence for Unit 1, and should be placed in your portfolio to show that you understand how to calculate face shapes. This will be important when you begin advising clients on the best hairstyle for them.

<aside>
Quick tip

Any experienced stylist will tell you that clients are not always realistic about what is possible. It is up to you to be positive and make alternative suggestions, rather than just saying that she can't have what she wants!
</aside>

Key Skills Activity Application of Number N2.1, N2.2, N2.3

With a tape measure:

1 Measure your face across the top of your cheekbones. Write down the measurement.

2 Now measure your jawline at the widest point. Write down the measurement.

3 Measure your forehead at the widest point; this will usually be halfway between your hairline and your eyebrows. Write down the measurement.

4 Measure from the tip of your hairline to the bottom of your chin. Write down the measurement.

Now for the clever part:

Oval: Length is equal to 1.5 times the width

Round: Face is as wide as it is long (or thereabouts)

Square: Face is as wide as it is long

Rectangular or long: Face is longer than it is wide

Heart shaped: Narrow at jaw line; wide at cheekbones and/or forehead

Diamond shaped: Widest at cheekbones, narrow forehead and jaw line of approximately equal widths

Pear shaped: Wide at jaw line and cheekbones but narrower at forehead.

Face shapes

Oval

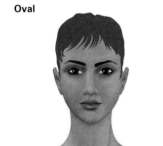

Round

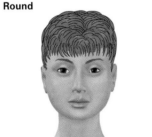

Square

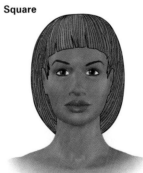

Rectangular

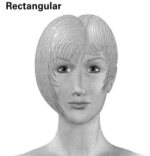

This face shape and bone structure is considered to be the ideal face shape. The chin tapers gently from a slightly wider forehead. Ideal for any hairstyle.

The face is usually short and broad with full cheeks and round contours. Width at the top of the head should be provided with height from the hair, which should be worn close at the sides.

The forehead is broad, corresponding with an angular jawline. This face shape should have a little height without width and the hair should taper well towards the jawline.

This face shape is narrow. Width is needed to shorten the face length. A fringe would be suitable with short hair. Asymmetric (unbalanced) styles also suit this face shape.

Heart shaped

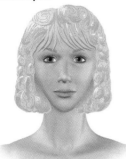

This shape usually has a wide forehead with the face tapering to a long jawline, rather like an inverted triangle. The aim of the hairstyle is to reduce the width across the forehead, emphasising the jawline.

Diamond shaped

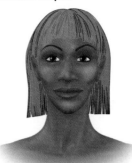

The forehead in this bone structure is narrow with the cheekbones extremely wide tapering to a narrow chin. The hairstyle should aim to minimise the width across the cheekbones. A central fringe should be worn with hair full below the cheeks but flat at the cheekbone line.

Pear shaped

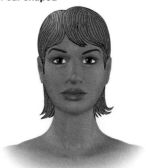

The forehead is narrow and the face gradually widens to the angle of the jaw, which is broad and prominent. The hairstyle should create the impression of width across the forehead and make the jawline seem narrower. The hair should be swept off the forehead to create an illusion of width with a reverse flicking fringe.

Quick tip

You will need to use all your tact to deal with situations when you are unable to carry out treatments, as the client may be embarrassed or angry. People sometimes act in unexpected ways to cover embarrassment or anger. The way you deal with the situation could mean the difference between a client who walks out of the salon and never comes back, and one who returns for treatments once her condition is cleared up.

Contraindications and scalp condition

Contraindications are any conditions that will limit the service that you can provide to the client. It is extremely important to discover if your client has any skin sensitivities, including any previous reactions to chemicals, or any medical conditions.

In the next unit, we will be looking in more detail at hair and scalp treatments, but you need to think about this at the consultation stage.

The chart on pages 93–95 in Unit 2 provides a list of scalp conditions – some of which are contagious. If you discover that a client has one of these contagious conditions, you will not be able to carry out any treatments in the salon until she has contacted her doctor or pharmacist and the condition has been cured.

The important things to remember are:

- ensure that your conversation with the client cannot be overheard by other clients in the salon
- explain what you have found clearly and calmly
- reassure the client that the condition can clear up with treatment
- advise the client about what she needs to do – for example, visit the doctor if the condition is ringworm, or buy a specialist preparation from the pharmacist if you have found head lice
- sterilise any brushes or tools that have been used on the client after she has left the salon
- clean the work area thoroughly using an anti-bacterial spray
- wash your hands carefully and thoroughly.

Key Skills Activity Communication C2.1a, C2.2 and C2.3

The following activity will provide excellent evidence for C2.1a. Ask the others in the group to sign witness statements to confirm that you took part in the discussion. If possible, ask a tutor to listen in to the discussion, and to assess your contribution.

Why not summarise the discussion afterwards, making sure that you include the points made by others as well as yourself, and provide evidence for C2.3 as well? This will not only give you valuable evidence, but it will also make you think about your discussion and reinforce the points raised.

Finally, you could obtain evidence for C2.2 by finding two different documents about this subject, and writing a short summary of the treatment for each condition. If you use images to illustrate your summary, you will have even more key skills evidence.

Group discussion:
Discuss the following scenarios with your group, and decide what you should do in each case:

1 Mrs Apple has psoriasis at the back of the ears. She requires a colour. What precautions will you have to take to ensure that the psoriasis is not irritated?

2 Mrs Pear is a regular client, and has severe eczema, which is apparent on the scalp. She gives you a doctor's note, stating that she can have chemicals applied directly to her scalp. Will you comply with her request for a root retouch?

3 Mrs Strawberry tells you during the consultation that she has used a blonde spray product on her hair. How can you find out if this product is compatible with other chemicals that you might need to use?

4 Mrs Plum is booked in for a semi-permanent colour. While you are helping her to select a colour, she mentions in passing that she had an allergic reaction to a colour in another salon. What would you do?

Hair texture, density, type, length and condition

The most valuable part of the consultation will be the visual checks that you carry out. You will need to consider the following factors.

The texture of the hair – How thick or fine is each individual hair? Is the hair fine, medium or thick? Texture may affect the porosity or elasticity of the hair. Hair may differ in texture throughout the hair length, and the points of the hair may be considerably finer. African Caribbean hair follows this pattern, and the fine points may break easily under heat or chemical treatments. Make sure that you take extra care, and carry out tests to ensure that you do not damage the hair.

The density (or volume) of hair – Remember, no two heads of hair are exactly the same. One client may have fine hair but lots of it, and another may have thick hair but little of it.

Fine hair has a small diameter, and tends to be light or weightless and flyaway. The hair is often straight and will not hold a curl very easily.

Medium hair is neither fine nor thick. It is the most common and most easily manageable type of hair.

Quick tip

This book could be used as one of your sources of evidence – now you only have to find one more!

(Remember we said in the introduction that key skills evidence can be gathered from activities that you carry out in the course of your diploma work, and that you should not have to do a lot of extra work. I hope that you are realising by now that this is true, and that you will start looking for other opportunities – you will probably find some that we have not highlighted.)

Hair texture

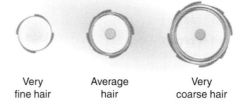

| Very
fine hair | Average
hair | Very
coarse hair |

Thick hair is wider in diameter and may be coarse. It feels rough and can lack shine. Thick hair is strong and can be hard to manage. It tends to be resistant to chemical processes.

You also need to establish the **hair type** that you are working with. There are three main types:

- Asian/Oriental – usually very straight with lots of cuticle scales for protection
- Caucasian/European – can be straight, wavy or curly
- African Caribbean – usually very tight curls.

Different hair types

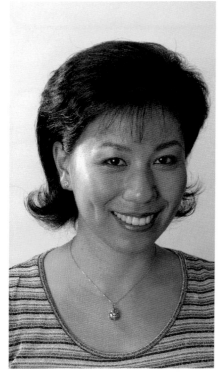

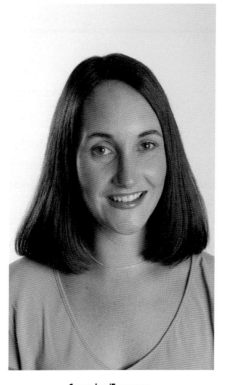

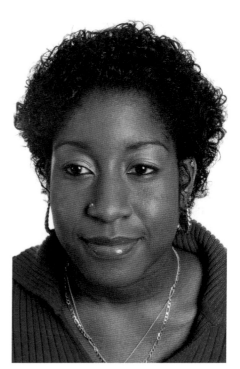

Asian/Oriental   **Caucasian/European**   **African Caribbean**

The length of the hair – Is the hair of one length? If it is, and it is long, it will have been shampooed and styled a great deal. It may have a build-up of chemical treatment on the older ends, which may affect the service that the client is requesting. On the other hand, is the hair long enough for the style the client wants? You may need to spend time guiding and growing the hair into the shape required, and in this case, you will have to consider how you (and the client) will manage the hair in the meantime.

The condition of the hair – Many factors will affect the condition of the hair, including:

- external factors – combing, brushing, shampooing, blow-drying, straightening, tonging and hair extensions
- weather – sun, wind, sea salt and extreme climates
- chemical effects – perming, bleaching, straightening, chlorine from swimming pools and salt from the sea
- general health and lifestyle – including effects of drugs, genetics, pregnancy, illness, operation side-effects, etc.

All these different factors will affect the condition of the hair. You will be able to assess condition by looking, feeling and, testing the hair, and by talking to the client. She will know if her hair is harder (or easier) to style than usual, and what particular problems she has been finding.

The hair test chart on the following page has some sections missing for you to fill in. See how you get on!

Remember that part of your job is to give your client advice on hair care. This can (and undoubtedly will) include advice on suitable products. It is also true, however, that a good balanced diet will contribute to good overall health, and this will be reflected in the hair and skin. It goes without saying that you will also practise what you preach!

Hair movement and growth patterns

To discover the hair's natural movement, you will need to see the hair in its natural state. When the hair is dry, it is difficult to recognise the natural fall of the hair, because of the styling aids and appliances that have been used. It is much easier to shampoo the hair first, comb it through and let the natural movement fall. This will help you to establish whether the hair is curly, wavy or naturally straight. You will also be able to analyse the hair to decide whether the client has any distinguishable growth patterns that may influence the choice of style.

The growth pattern means the direction that the hair grows from the root.

On some people, growth patterns are very obvious and apparent; on others, you may need to part the hair to look for the direction in which the hair is growing.

	Purpose of test	Method	Expected result	When to do the test	Potential consequences of not carrying out the test
Elasticity test	To determine hair strength	Stretch one or two hairs between fingers and thumbs			
Porosity test	To determine the condition of the cuticle		Hair should feel smooth		Damage to the hair. This could result in potential legal action
Incompatibility test		Mix 1 part perm lotion to 20 parts hydrogen peroxide, place cutting in solution and leave for 30 minutes		Before any chemical process	
Skin test	To test for any skin or scalp allergies				
Strand test			The colour may need further development time		The result may not meet requirements. Damage to the hair may occur, which could lead to client taking legal action
Development test for perming	To find out if the perm is developed				

Hair test chart

There are some different growth patterns to consider, as shown below.

Cowlick – This is usually found in the front hairline. This may cause problems if the client requires a very straight fringe. You may need to make the fringe heavier to encourage the weight to hold it down. This is best cut freehand on dry hair.

Widow's peak – This is found at the centre of the front hairline. The hairline grows to an obvious point. Again, this can cause problems if the client wants a fringe. You will need to cut it freehand on dry hair.

Double crown – As the name suggests, the client will have two crown partings. They may be joined, or there may be a gap in between. This growth pattern is easy to identify on short hair, but it is harder to spot on longer hair. If it is not obvious, you need to part the hair to discover the growth pattern, as this may influence your choice of style.

Quick tip

The main rule with a double crown is not to cut the hair too short at the crown, or it will stick up!

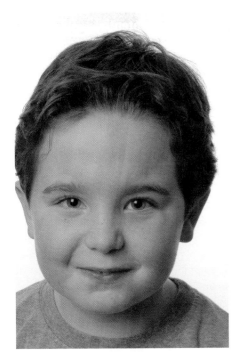

Cowlick

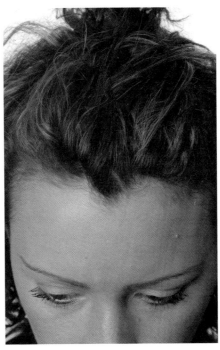

Widow's peak

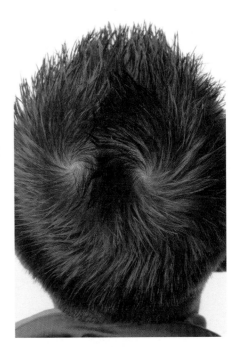

Double crown

Nape whorl – This is when the hairline around the nape area grows unevenly. The hair may not lay flat in this area if it is cut too short. Usually the hair at the nape grows into the middle creating a 'whorl'. This growth pattern has a number of nicknames that you will come to know from experience in the hairdressing industry. You need to ensure when cutting short hair that enough weight is left to help keep it flat. The alternative is to cut very short using the clipper/scissor-over-comb technique to ensure neatness is achieved on the hairline.

Hair growth cycle – The word **ACT** will help you remember the order of the growth cycle:

A = Anagen
C = Catagen
T = Telogen

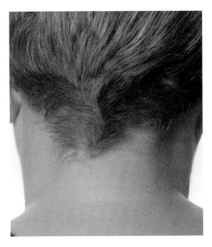

Nape whorl

Anagen is the active growing stage, which may last between one and seven years. This will differ with each individual. Some clients cannot grow their hair past their shoulders, whilst others will grow it to reach their waist. At this stage, the formation at the base of the follicle is apparent. This will determine the hair's thickness, shape, texture and colour. Around 80–90 per cent of our scalp hairs will be in this stage at any one time.

Catagen is the breakdown and changing stage which will last for about two weeks. During this short time, the follicles undergo a period of change and do not grow. However, new cells are forming. The hair bulb gradually separates from the papilla and moves further up the follicle. Only one per cent of the follicles will be in the catagen stage at any one time.

Telogen is the resting and final stage which will last for around three–four months. During this period, the follicle begins to shrink and separates itself from the papilla area. Towards the end of this stage, new cells begin to activate in preparation for the new anagen stage of regrowth. If the old hair is still in the follicle, the new hair will push it out. About 13 per cent of the follicles will be in this stage at any one time.

The hair growth cycle

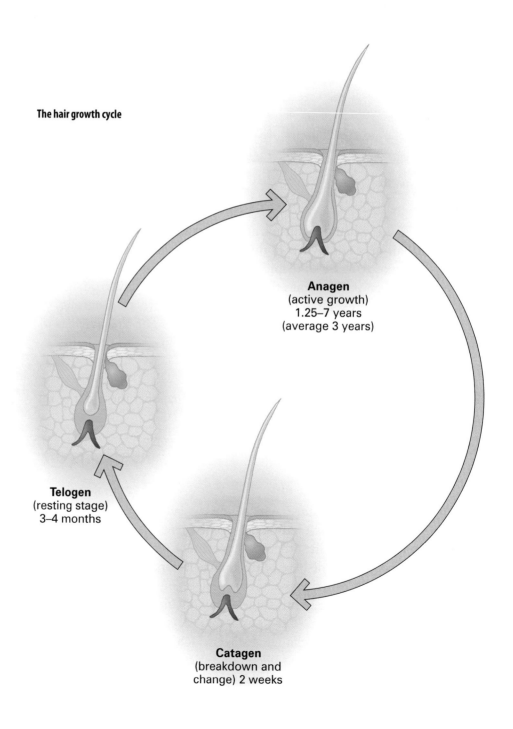

Anagen
(active growth)
1.25–7 years
(average 3 years)

Telogen
(resting stage)
3–4 months

Catagen
(breakdown and
change) 2 weeks

Client's lifestyle, body shape and features

Lifestyle – Your client's lifestyle will influence the choice of style that she can achieve and maintain. Remember that she will need a hairstyle that she can manage.

Quite often, clients have a firm idea of the look they want; they may even bring a picture to show their ideas. In this case, you should discuss the suitability of this style for your client's hair type. You may need to offer some suggestions about how the style could be adapted to suit her hair type, face shape or lifestyle. Even if the style seems completely unsuited to your client, you will probably be able to find some elements of it that could be incorporated into a new style.

It is up to you to ask some simple questions.
- How long can she spend on her hair each day?
- Does she find it easy to style her own hair?
- Can she afford the maintenance, such as colour retouching?

You will also need to take your client's personality into account. You don't want to send a shy, introverted client out with an eccentric, whacky hairstyle.

The age of the client may also be a factor. Younger clients may be more likely to try a different style, whereas older clients may tend to stick to the same style. Perhaps a change of style would boost a client's morale and make her appear younger? Clients might appreciate some suggestions, as long as they are not too way-out! Don't forget that two people can be the same age, and one can appear much younger because of the way they dress and their personalities.

Remember that the client's job may need to be taken into account. For example, clients with the following occupations may have specific requirements.
- Operating machinery – The hair may need to be tied back off the face or kept short.
- Model – May need a specific look, but will probably need a versatile style.
- Nurse, cook or food handler – For reasons of hygiene, the hair may need to be tied up or kept off the face.
- Flight attendant – Will need to look smart, and may wear a hat as part of the uniform.
- Businesswoman – Will want to look smart, practical and not too fussy.
- Army, navy, air force or police personnel – The hair will need to be short and neat, or long enough to tie up. A hat will also be worn as part of the uniform.

Quick tip

Beware of the client who just says 'I want something different and I'll leave it to you. Do whatever you think.' Clients rarely mean it! Make sure that you discuss the options with her, and agree what you are going to do. This will give you both more confidence about the whole procedure!

Some occupations may have specific style requirements

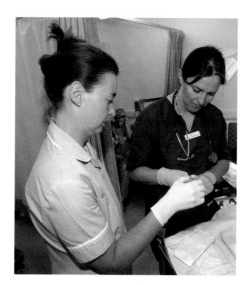

Nurse

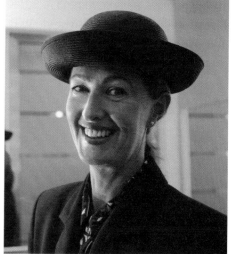

Flight attendant

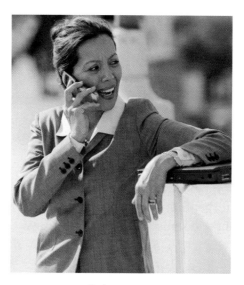

Businesswoman

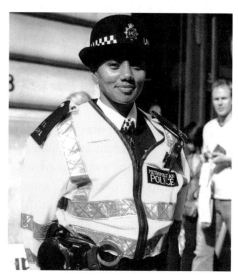

Police officer

Portfolio Activity

A new client comes into the salon, and asks for advice on a suitable hair style.

She tells you that she has two young children aged three and five, and is about to return to work as a nurse. She is fairly slim, but has a round face. Her hair is fine and straight, and lacks body. She tells you that her hair goes flat by the end of the day, and she washes and blow dries it every morning in an attempt to give it some 'bounce'. Her hair is shoulder length, with split, uneven ends.

Look through a variety of magazines, and select some suitable hairstyles for this client. Write a short report explaining why you have chosen each style, and point out the benefits for the client bearing in mind her lifestyle and occupation.

Body shape – Your aim should be to make sure that the hairstyle will flatter the client. For example, an extremely short and spiky hair cut would not be the best choice for a tall, very slim client. Why is this?

Features – You will need to assess the client's features to ensure that you enhance the good features and detract the eye from those that are not so flattering. There are different ways to do this, as shown below.

- A prominent, large nose will be diminished if you can create softness around the hairline. Avoid centre partings and keep hair swept back off the face. A fringe should be full and loose, not flat to the head.
- Low or high foreheads can be disguised by adding fringes.
- Square or prominent jawlines can be disguised by creating softness at the sides and keeping some length. Choose a style that clings to the jawline. Fringes will help balance the shape.
- Double chins require length and softness. Add some height to balance the look.
- Protruding ears are best covered. For men you can leave the hair touching the top of the ears and leave sideburns to help create length in this area.
- If the client wears glasses you will need to take this into account. It is often best to discourage too much hair around the face, in order to show the client's other features as well. If the hair is on the face and then glasses are added, the look can be 'crowded'.
- Long, thin necks need to be softened around the jawline. Avoid one-length haircuts, and also avoid height.
- Short, wide necks need to be disguised by adding height and avoiding hairstyles that are too short or too long.
- High or receding foreheads needs to be softened by adding full fringes and avoiding height above the forehead.

If you have an accurate vision in your head of what you are going to create, taking into account all the above facts, your client is likely to feel at ease and comfortable with the advice you have given. If you try to rush the consultation, your client will sense this, and will inevitably be uneasy and uncomfortable.

A rushed consultation is likely to lead to an unsatisfactory result and a dissatisfied client. You will probably have to spend even more time trying to put matters right than you would have spent conducting a proper consultation in the first place. More to the point, the client is unlikely to return and you will have lost business for your salon.

Quick tip

A full consultation on a new client should be completed within 10 to 15 minutes. The consultation will help determine the success of the service.

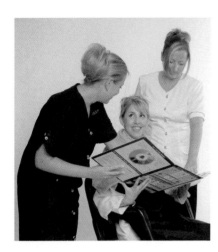

Make sure your client is clear about what the treatment is likely to involve

Clarify your understanding

After the consultation, and before you start work on your client, make sure that you are both clear about what you have agreed! It might be useful to use photographs from magazines or catalogues to illustrate suggestions that you make.

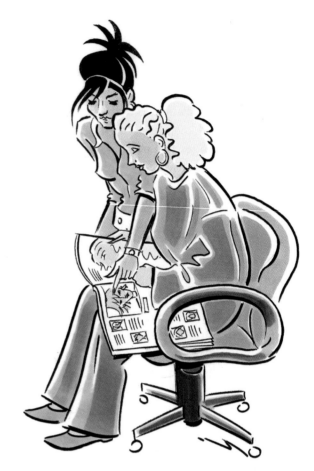

Photos in magazines can help you and your client to make sure that you both have the same idea in mind!

Recommend after-care procedures and additional salon services

Sale of products to clients

The sale of products has become increasingly important in hairdressing salons. Gone are the days when the only items for sale on the reception desk were rain hats and plastic combs.

There are several reasons why the sale of a product can be a good thing.
- It makes a contribution to the income of the salon.
- It provides a service to clients, who do not have to go to another shop to make their purchases.

- Hairdressers can recommend suitable products to help the client maintain her hairstyle between visits. If clients find their style is easy to manage, they are likely to return.
- Clients might feel more confident about purchasing relatively expensive products if these have been recommended by their hairdresser than if they were buying in a chemist or supermarket.

So, how do you go about selling products to your clients?

The first thing to remember is that clients are buying advice as well as a product. If you sell them something that does not suit their hair type, or which does not do what you promised, they won't buy again. What's more, they might not even return to the salon. This means that you need to think very carefully about every sale you make.

Display

Shopkeepers spend a great deal of time ensuring that their goods are displayed attractively because they know that this will lead to sales. Take a tip from them!

Imagine that you are a client. If you walked into a salon and found a grubby display stand containing an assortment of dusty bottles, with no prices displayed, and no indication of what each product was for, would you be tempted to buy? Probably not!

However, if you found a gleaming display unit containing well-displayed products in clean bottles, with prices clearly shown, you would probably be more inclined to buy, especially if a helpful hairdresser could offer you informed advice about which products were most suitable for you.

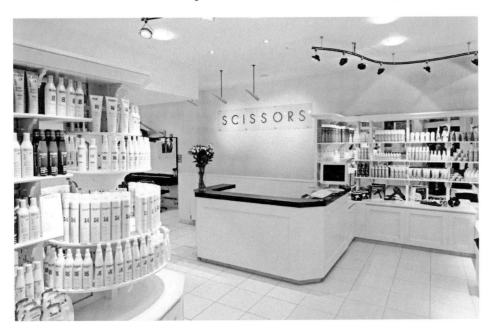

Retail product displays must look attractive to tempt clients to buy

Consider this

In your salon, who is responsible for ensuring that the display stand is clean and properly stocked?

What would you do if you noticed that some products had sold out?

Advice

Your clients can buy shampoo, conditioner and all types of hair products with their weekly grocery shop at the supermarket. One reason they will buy from your salon instead is that they can get expert advice about the best products for them.

A good time to give advice is during the client's treatment. If you explain why you are using a particular product, the client may well buy some for use at home. In addition, asking if they have had problems with their hair could give you the opportunity to recommend a suitable treatment.

If your salon has a receptionist who is not a hairdresser, it is important that they consult the stylist who has served the client before making any recommendations. However well the receptionist knows the stock, it is the stylist who knows the client's hair!

Portfolio Activity

Consider the products you stock in your salon, then think about what advice you would give in the following cases.

1 It is winter, and a client with fine, straight hair tells you that her hair has static electricity which makes it difficult to manage. Is there anything she can do about this?

2 A client has blonde highlights put in for the first time and asks you if she will need to use a different shampoo and/or conditioner. What advice would you give?

3 Your client tells you that she is about to leave on a trip to the Caribbean. What advice would you give her about hair care during her holiday?

4 A client asks you to suggest a suitable conditioner for her daughter but you have never seen the daughter. What questions would you ask, and what recommendations would you make?

Key Skills Activity Communication C2.1b, C2.3

You could use the information you have gathered for the above portfolio activity to give a talk to your group about the products you stock in your salon, and what they should be used for. Make the talk about four minutes long. When you give the talk, speak clearly in a way that suits your subject, purpose and situation (2.1b.1). Keep to the subject and structure the talk so that your group follows what you are saying (2.1b.2). Use appropriate ways of supporting your main points, such as photographs or samples (2.1b.3).

While we're on the subject of Communication key skills, why not write a short newsletter for your salon's clients on the subject of the products you sell. Give advice on what they should be used for? Perhaps your manager would agree to this being given to clients?

Making a sale

If you have made sure that your products are displayed well and have given good advice to your clients, then you have already started to make a sale. However, you must also remember that customers are protected by various laws when they buy anything from your salon, so you have to make sure that you do not contravene any of the legislation.

Quick tip

No doubt you have spotted that the information you gather for the first of the activities above could also be used to provide data for the second.

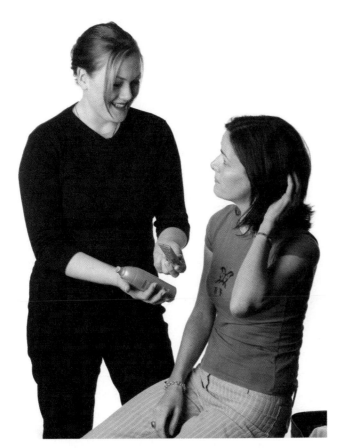

Good advice to your client on what is best for her hair can help to make a sale

Legislation

Trade Descriptions Act 1987

Under this Act, it is an offence to make an untrue or exaggerated claim about goods being offered for sale. For example, if your client, John, is losing his hair, you must not tell him that a particular shampoo will make his hair grow back unless you are positive that it will do so. (If you really do have a shampoo that will guarantee hair growth, you are well on your way to making your first million!)

If you make false claims, your customer is entitled to complain to the Trading Standards Department. Quite apart from the fact that a hefty fine could be imposed, your salon could receive very unwelcome publicity in local newspapers!

Sale of Goods Act 1979 and Supply of Goods Act 1994

This legislation ensures that consumers are protected if the goods or services they buy are faulty, or do not meet their reasonable requirements.

Goods must be fit for the purpose for which they are sold, of reasonable quality, and meet any claims made for them.

Services must be provided at a reasonable price, within a reasonable time and to a reasonable standard.

Your customers are entitled to expect that anything they buy will be:
- in good condition, fit for normal use and not faulty
- fit for the purpose for which it is sold; this means that John would be able to complain if the shampoo did not make his hair grow again
- as described; for example, a plastic make-up bag must not be sold as 'leather'.

If the goods or services provided do not meet this legislation, the customer is entitled to a refund of the price paid. However, this Act only applies to faulty goods. It does not apply if the customer changes his or her mind about the goods.

Consumer Protection Act 1987

There are three sections to this Act.
- **Unsafe goods** – It is a criminal offence to sell goods which are unsafe. Your customers are entitled to expect that anything they buy from you will meet all relevant safety levels. For example, if your salon offers hairdryers for sale, they must meet electrical safety standards. If the hairdryers are of a reputable make, purchased from an established wholesaler, and meet British Standards, you can offer them for sale with reasonable confidence. Traders who sell unsafe goods could be fined or imprisoned.

- **Misleading information or suggestions** – It is illegal for a retailer to mislead customers about prices. You should display a current list of VAT-inclusive prices.
- **Product liability** – If a product does not meet the standard that the customer is reasonably entitled to expect, it is faulty. If a faulty product causes injury or death, your customer or her dependants could claim compensation.

Consider this

Your boss arrived at the salon on Monday morning carrying a boxful of hairdryers that he had bought at a car boot sale the previous day. The dryers do not have plugs fitted, and you have never heard of the manufacturer.

Make a list of your reasons for *not* offering the dryers for sale. Include information about any relevant legislation.

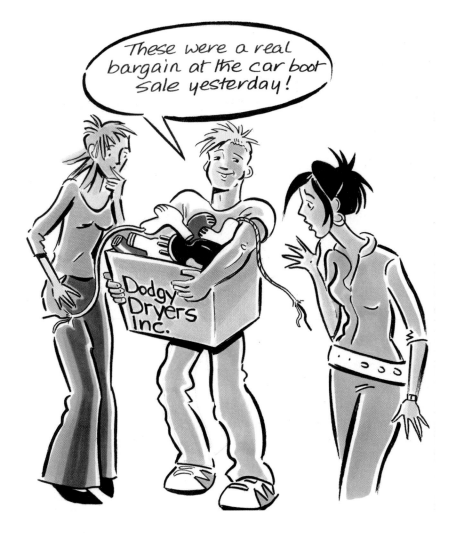

What would you do about these?

Notices displayed by retailers who are attempting to 'opt out' of legislation have no effect. In the past, before consumer legislation was introduced, it was not unusual to see notices such as:

> # NO REFUNDS MADE
> # ON ANY PRODUCTS
> # FOR ANY REASON

In these more enlightened times, customers can safely ignore such notices!

The legislation applies to all goods, including those sold at reduced prices. The only exception to this is if a product had a fault which was pointed out to the customer at the time of sale. In such a case, the customer could not claim a refund because of that fault. However, her rights are unaffected if other faults become apparent.

For example, if a customer bought a hairbrush which was reduced because the box was damaged, she could claim a refund if the bristles fell out within a couple of days.

Key Skills Activity Communication C2.1a

Don't forget that all group discussions offer key skills Communication evidence.

Group discussion:

This is an exercise for you to carry out with the rest of your group. You also need to put yourself in the customer's place.

You have bought a pack of hair products which the receptionist recommended for your blonde hair. On reaching home, you find that the shampoo bottle is split and has leaked over all the other products. When you read the small print on the back of the pack you notice that the products are recommended for brunettes.

You return to the salon, and ask for a refund.

The receptionist points to a notice that says 'No refunds made for any reason'.

1 In your group, make a list of the legislation that offers you protection in this case.

2 If the receptionist had pointed out the leaking bottle at the time of sale, and had given you 25 per cent discount, how would this affect your rights?

3 What effect do you think the salon's attitude might have on its customers? Would you use the salon again if it treated you like this?

Key Skills Activity Communication C2.2

Other members of staff who sell your salon's products might not be aware of the Acts to which they are subject. Choose one of the Acts mentioned above and, using at least two different sources (one of which could be this book), summarise the main points contained in it (and perhaps think about the reasons for them). Then write a document summarising the information for your colleagues. Make the document at least 500 words long.

Communicating with clients

Have you ever thought about how many different types of communication you use every day?

Consider this

Make a list of the communication methods you use. My list is given in the spider diagram below. Can you think of any methods that I have missed?

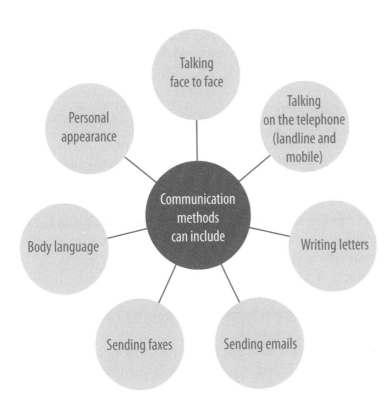

Communication methods

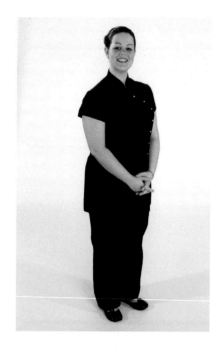

**Good personal presentation gives
a positive image**

Personal appearance

Some of these communication methods might have surprised you. Is personal appearance really a method of communication? Yes! Your non-verbal communication includes your personal presentation and body language (see below) and will say more about you than your words can.

Imagine this: You walk into a shop and see the shop assistant slouching in a corner. Her hair is dirty, her nails are filthy, she is wearing a stained and dirty overall, her shoes are scuffed and muddy, and her tights are laddered. She is communicating a message to you without even opening her mouth and the message is: 'I don't care what I look like, I don't have any self-respect, and I don't care enough about my customers to bother to come to work looking decent'.

As a hairdresser, you are working closely with people and providing a very personal service. Your clients come to you because they want to look good and they won't have much confidence in your ability to improve their appearance if you can't manage your own. Check out the personal appearance checklist opposite.

Body language

Closely aligned with personal appearance is body language.

Did you know that we make up our minds about people within 20 seconds of meeting them (even before they have opened their mouth). We make hundreds of subconscious judgements and decisions and arrive at a 'gut reaction' feeling.

It is quite unnerving to think that you could alienate people without meaning to, so let's look at the sort of signals you send out.

- **Facial expression** – Everybody responds to a genuine smile. Note the word 'genuine'. A false smile fools nobody and can be as off-putting as a scowl.
- **Posture** – Somebody who stands or sits straight and holds her head up high will look confident even if she is not feeling it. On the other hand, somebody who slouches may look unsure (or even furtive).
- **Eye contact** – It would be unnerving to speak to somebody who stared you in the eye the whole time. However, if somebody refuses to meet your eyes at all, you may suspect that she is trying to hide something or is not telling the whole truth.
- **Gestures** – Fiddling with rings, twitching, blinking, wringing hands or crossing arms are all gestures that can indicate nervousness, self-defence or insecurity.

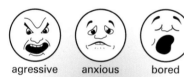
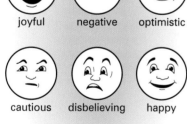
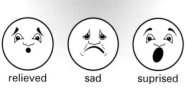

agressive   anxious   bored

joyful   negative   optimistic

cautious   disbelieving   happy

relieved   sad   suprised

Facial expressions

PERSONAL APPEARANCE CHECKLIST

Hair	You won't be a very good ambassador for your salon if your own hair is a mess! Whatever style you choose, your hair must be clean and well-groomed. If you have long hair, make sure that it is styled so that it does not hang over your client's face when you are shampooing. Unless you work for a very trendy salon, your boss might prefer it if you kept your whackier styles for nights out!
Skin and make-up	Clean, well-cared for skin is essential. No amount of make-up can compensate for this! Again, unless you work for a trendy salon, you might prefer to keep your wilder flights of fancy for clubbing nights. If you work for a salon which caters for a young, trendy clientele, you might set trends with your make-up. On the other hand, clients at a more traditional salon might not be happy if you appear with fantastic make-up and piercings.
Hands and nails	Your hands are on show, and come into contact with your clients! It goes without saying that your hands and nails should be scrupulously clean at all times. Remember that long nails and large rings can scratch your clients when you are carrying out treatments, so shorter nails and few rings are probably the order of the day.
Clothing	Some hairdressers wear a uniform or have a dress code, some wear an overall and others wear their own choice of clothes. Whatever you wear, the important thing is that it is clean and well-pressed. Shoes should be comfortable, as you will be on your feet all day. They should also be clean. Tights must have no holes or ladders — it's a good idea to keep a spare pair in your bag! If you wear open-toed shoes, you run the risk of getting hair splinters in your feet. This can be very painful, and could lead to infections.
Personal hygiene	It goes without saying (we hope!) that you will take care of your personal hygiene. This means regular bathing or showering and using a good deodorant, cleaning your teeth morning, night and after lunch, and avoiding heavy, cloying scents. Imagine what would happen if half a dozen stylists all wore different, heavy scents. Pity the poor clients!
Jewellery	Water and product can get trapped under rings, and this can lead to contact dermatitis. This is not only unpleasant and unsightly, but it could even result in your having to give up hairdressing.

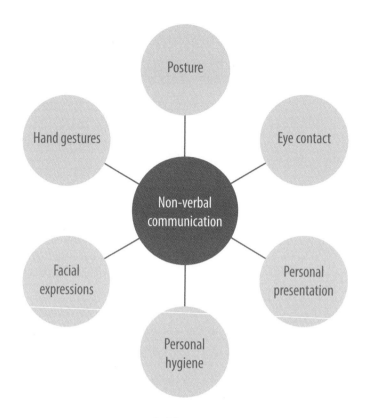

Body language

Body language can be positive or negative. How good are you at deciphering it?

Consider this

Look at the following types of body language. Which of them are positive and which are negative?

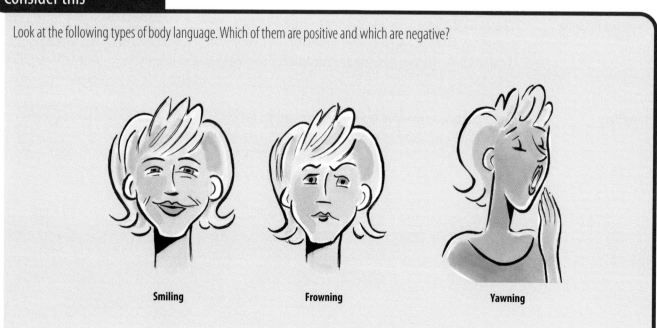

Smiling   Frowning   Yawning

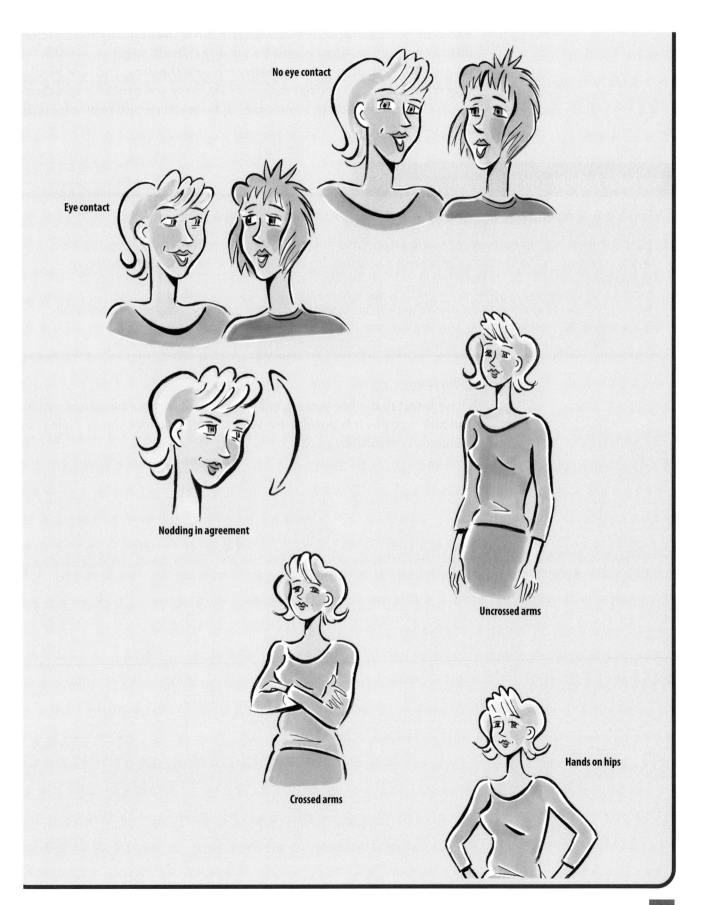

No eye contact

Eye contact

Nodding in agreement

Uncrossed arms

Crossed arms

Hands on hips

The main point about body language is that it is unconscious and extremely difficult to disguise. Most people find it very difficult to get away with telling a lie. No matter how much they rehearse the story, and how hard they try to sound convincing, their body language will probably give them away. Confidence tricksters know this and work very hard to control their body language.

Key Skills Activity Communication C2.1a

This is a group discussion exercise for you to do with the rest of your group. You will need about five people.

Each person needs to think of two true statements about themselves and one untrue statement. The members of the group then take it in turns to stand up in front of the others and make the three statements. The group then has to decide which of the statements are true and which are false.

When it is your turn, try as hard as you can to control your body language so that you do not give yourself away. You will probably find this very hard to do!

Talking face to face

Don't forget that when you are talking, you will be communicating verbally and non-verbally. It is possible for your words to say one thing, while your gestures say something else!

Word search 1

The following words, which relate to the structure of the skin, are contained in the word search grid. Circle each of the words in the grid. Words run horizontally, vertically, diagonally and backwards.

EPIDERMIS	SEBACEOUS	FOLLICLE	BLOOD SUPPLY
PAPILLA	SWEAT	HORNY	BULB
DERMIS	ARRECTOR PILI	HAIR SHAFT	PRICKLE
GRANULAR			

E	P	I	M	I	S	P	A	P	I	S	E	B	A	C	H
A	I	R	D	H	E	I	N	P	A	P	B	K	E	L	L
Y	E	P	I	D	E	R	M	I	S	N	E	U	W	E	S
L	L	O	L	I	V	A	P	P	A	P	I	L	L	A	I
E	R	B	L	O	O	E	L	K	C	I	R	P	D	B	M
S	U	P	P	Y	L	L	G	G	R	A	N	U	L	A	R
H	E	S	E	B	A	C	E	O	U	S	I	N	E	M	E
A	N	W	N	B	R	H	E	N	D	A	L	E	D	O	D
N	A	E	R	D	J	F	O	L	L	I	C	L	E	O	A
N	N	A	E	I	L	I	P	R	O	T	C	E	R	R	A
K	E	T	V	I	N	H	O	R	N	Y	O	L	M	I	V
H	A	I	R	S	H	A	F	T	E	R	P	E	A	N	G
B	L	O	O	D	S	U	P	P	L	Y	R	E	L	S	F
O	R	D	B	E	R	V	E	E	N	D	H	A	I	F	G
L	L	H	A	E	X	Z	C	M	D	E	R	T	U	M	N
T	U	S	I	A	R	R	P	I	L	B	U	B	P	I	C

Word search 2

This grid contains words that relate to the structure of the skull. Circle each of the following words in the grid. Words run horizontally, vertically, diagonally and backwards.

PARIETAL
SUTURES
MANDIBLE

NASAL
ZYGOMATIC

TEMPORAL
MAXILLA

OCCIPITAL
FRONTAL

P	A	R	I	S	U	T	U	M	A	X	I	L	L	A	P
U	N	M	R	I	E	E	M	P	O	R	A	L	P	A	R
I	E	T	S	U	T	E	R	K	E	L	L	H	E	I	N
E	E	M	A	N	N	B	R	E	N	D	A	Y	N	A	S
L	A	P	A	R	I	E	T	A	L	H	A	I	D	O	R
B	S	Z	S	I	N	G	N	V	Q	H	E	I	C	N	E
I	A	N	Y	K	S	U	T	U	R	E	S	C	E	F	L
D	N	E	W	G	E	N	A	S	A	L	I	L	L	R	R
N	T	E	M	P	O	R	A	L	N	P	D	A	L	O	O
A	A	R	D	O	L	M	A	X	I	L	L	X	I	N	E
M	J	O	A	N	N	L	A	T	E	I	R	A	P	T	K
E	V	I	N	P	E	N	A	T	G	R	E	S	F	A	R
D	H	E	I	N	E	L	M	A	I	N	N	T	E	L	P
O	E	O	C	C	I	P	Z	Y	G	C	P	A	R	I	X
I	L	L	A	M	T	O	R	A	L	E	M	P	H	A	I
R	G	D	M	R	O	E	D	S	E	S	R	I	N	A	P

Portfolio Activity

Can you replace the numbers on the following diagram of a skull with the names of the bones?

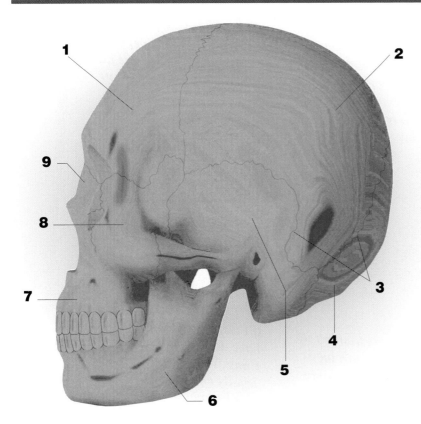

1 _____

2 _____

3 _____

4 _____

5 _____

6 _____

7 _____

8 _____

9 _____

Consultation Know How

1 What are the six facts that should be considered during a consultation?

2 What is meant by contraindications?

3 What are the three different textures of hair?

4 List at least three factors that contribute to the condition of the hair.

5 What are the three stages of the hair growth cycle?

6 List some occupations that may influence your client's choice of hairstyle.

7 How long should a full consultation take to complete?

8 Give three reasons why the sale of a product is a good thing.

9 What are the names of the Acts that you must comply with when selling goods?

10 Why is it a good idea to change stock display stands regularly?

Kelly's Problem Page

Dear Kelly

I purchased a hairbrush from my local hair salon, but when I got it home, I changed my mind. When I took it back, the salon refused to refund my money or change it. Surely I have rights under the Sale of Goods Act?

Kelly replies:

No, I'm afraid the Sale of Goods Act does not cover this situation, as the brush was not faulty. You are not entitled to a refund or an exchange just because you change your mind. After all, what would the salon do with the brush when you took it back? They couldn't sell it to anybody else. Would you want to buy a brush that somebody else had taken home and used?

Dear Kelly

My boss asked me to mark up the prices on some products and put them on the display stand. I made a mistake and marked some conditioner at £3.99 instead of £7.99. I realised this when a customer brought some to the cash desk and when I charged her £7.99 she said that she was entitled to have it for £3.99. I refused to sell it to her and she made an awful fuss. In the end, my boss came out and said she could have it for £3.99 and then made me change all the prices on the ones on the stand. I'm really annoyed with my boss for making me look silly in front of the customer.

Kelly replies:

If I were your boss, I would have done exactly the same thing. Your customer was not legally entitled to buy the conditioner at the cheaper price, because a marked price is what is called an 'offer to treat' which just means an offer to trade. If you had noticed the mistake after you had taken the customer's money, you would have made a contract with her and you could not then have asked her for more money.

Your boss was not trying to make you look silly, she was just trying to keep a customer happy. It is easy to lose customers and very hard to regain them, so your boss probably thought it was better to sell at the lower price than to risk losing a customer.

Your Notes

Your Notes

UNIT8

CONTRIBUTE TO MAINTAINING HEALTH, SAFETY AND SECURITY OF THE SALON ENVIRONMENT

Introduction

Health and safety is important in every workplace, but if you think about the problems that could arise in a salon, you will appreciate that it is absolutely essential that you follow health and safety procedures to the letter.

You could be the best hairdresser in the country, but if you are not operating in accordance with health and safety requirements, you will be putting yourself, your clients and other staff at serious risk. You will not learn how to cut, style, perm or colour hair in this unit, but you will learn how to do all these things safely.

In this unit you will learn how to:
- support emergency procedures
- support and maintain health, safety and security at work.

This unit also relates to other Hairdressing National Occupational Standards:

Level 2 Unit 209 – Support the health, safety and security of the salon environment
Levels 2 and 3 Unit G1 – Ensure your own actions reduce risks to health and safety.

You will produce evidence from simulations and from your workplace, such as witness testimonies and product evidence. For example, if you take part in a fire drill in the salon, you should write down exactly what you did and ask your boss to sign it.

You will also take a short, externally marked written test covering the underpinning knowledge requirements of this important unit.

Support emergency procedures

Everybody hopes that emergencies will never arise in the workplace and most of the time they don't.

It is precisely because emergencies occur so rarely that they need to be thought about and planned for. In contrast, the telephone probably rings all the time in your salon so you will get lots of practice in answering it, taking messages and making bookings. You do it all the time and you are, we hope, confident that you can do it properly.

You might not be quite so confident about how you would act in the event of an emergency, such as a fire in the salon. If it happens, you will need to know exactly what to do, but you cannot practise under 'real' conditions, so you will have to use simulations.

You should also be familiar with your salon's health and safety policies and procedures. These will probably cover the different aspects shown in the diagram below.

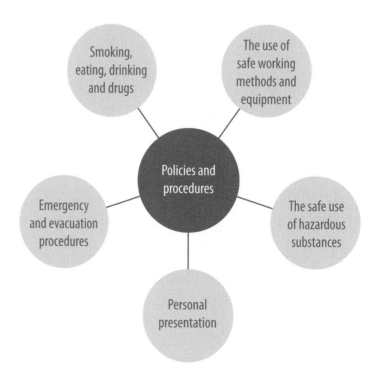

Workplace health and safety policies and procedures

You will probably have been given a copy of your salon's health and safety policy and if not, you should ask for one. Read through the policy and put a copy into your portfolio.

What procedure is specified in the event of a fire?

Fire procedures

Fire procedures will differ from salon to salon but they will all have the same aims.

- To raise the alarm.
- To get everybody to safety and account for them.
- To call the emergency services.
- To prevent the fire from spreading.
- To minimise the damage to property.

If you discovered a fire in the stock room of your salon, how would you raise the alarm? Is there a break-glass alarm? Where is it situated?

An outline of a typical fire procedure might be as follows.

1 On discovering a fire, raise the alarm. Fire alarm points are situated in the kitchen, the reception area, the stock room and the basin area. A very small fire may be tackled with the appropriate fire extinguisher, but only if it is safe to do so. *Do not put yourself at risk*. Raise the alarm before trying to tackle a fire, however small.

2 On hearing the alarm, staff should take their clients out of the building and everybody should congregate in the car park at the front of the salon.

3 The receptionist should dial 999 and ask for the Fire Service. The receptionist should take the appointments book and visitors' book on leaving the salon.

4 Each stylist is responsible for ensuring that her clients leave the salon.

5 The fire marshals for each floor will check that their areas are clear. (NB: the fire marshals should be named and staff should be aware of who they are.)

6 Once outside, the manager will take a roll-call of staff and clients.

7 Nobody must re-enter the building until permission has been given by the manager and/or emergency services.

8 Raising the alarm is vital and should be done as soon as a fire is discovered. Even a few seconds could be vital and none of the other procedures will take place until the alarm has been raised.

Every organisation should have named fire marshals. In practice, in a small salon there might be only one, but in a larger salon there should be one for each floor at least. The marshals are responsible for ensuring that everybody gets out of the building safely in the event of a fire. You should follow their instructions.

Fire drills

Every workplace should have regular fire drills and staff should know what the fire alarm sounds like, what they have to do when they hear it, and where they have to meet outside the salon. You might groan when your boss holds a fire drill (especially if it's raining at the time) but if a genuine emergency should arise, you will be relieved that you have practised the procedure and that you know exactly what to do. Everyone is far more likely to keep calm and less likely to panic if they know what they need to do and are confident that they can do it.

Remember, you need to think of your clients as well as yourself, and they may be frightened and inclined to panic. They will look to you to deal with the situation, and a calm but firm approach is what is needed.

Remember: panic is contagious!

Fire-fighting equipment

Your salon should be equipped with fire extinguishers. They should be mounted on walls on special brackets, and should not be free-standing. This should ensure that you always know where they are if you need them. The following chart shows the different types of extinguisher and what each should be used for.

Type of fire	Water extinguisher	Foam spray	ABC powder	Carbon dioxide (CO_2)
Wood Paper Textiles	Yes	Yes	Yes	
Flammable liquids		Yes	Yes	Yes
Gaseous fires			Yes	Yes
Live electrical equipment			Yes	Yes

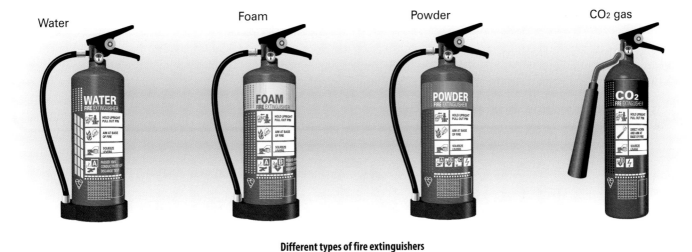

Different types of fire extinguishers

Portfolio Activity

1 Draw a plan of your salon (one for each floor, if the salon is on more than one level).

2 Mark on the plan the position of all fire alarms and fire extinguishers. Show what type of fire each extinguisher can be used for, and write the date on which the extinguisher was last checked. You will find this information somewhere on the extinguisher.

3 Draw another plan of the outside of the salon, showing the place where everybody should congregate in the event of a fire.

4 Finally, write down the names of the fire marshals.

First aid

However careful people are, accidents can happen. If somebody is hurt, he or she might require first aid, but remember, first aid is just what it says. It is the first thing you do *before* calling for professional help, if necessary.

There should be a qualified first aider in your salon who should be called if anybody has an accident. This person will have been trained to use basic procedures and will also know when to call for medical help.

If somebody has an accident, do not rush in and try to help if you don't know what you are doing. You could do more harm than good. Always call for the first aider.

Your salon will also have a first aid box and it should be somebody's job to make sure that it contains the correct supplies.

Quick tip

Make sure you know the name of the first aider at work. Find out now – don't wait until somebody has had an accident.

Portfolio Activity

1 Where is your salon's first aid box stored?

2 Find the box and list the contents making sure that none of them is out of date.

3 Write down the name(s) of the first aider(s) in your salon.

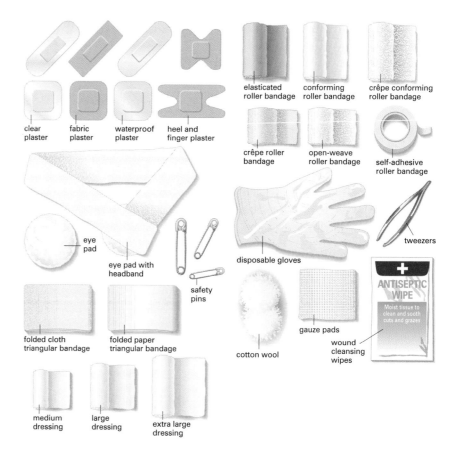

Items for a first aid box

You might like to become a first aider yourself. Ask your boss if you can take a course. These last for four days (for a qualified first aider) or one day (for an assistant).

Accident book

Your salon should also have an accident book in which *all* accidents, however small, are entered.

Portfolio Activity

1 Speak to the first aider in your salon and find out the correct procedure for dealing with the following incidents:

   a) A child, Maryam Ali, slips on the floor of the salon and bangs her head. A large bump appears. You see it happen.

   b) A stylist, Jane Stone, cuts her finger when cutting a client's hair. The cut is not deep, but is bleeding. A colleague, Charlotte Brown, is with her at the time.

   c) Charlotte Brown faints when she sees Jane's cut. Charlotte is four months' pregnant.

   d) A client, Wesley Lewis, has an epileptic fit. Your manager, Marc Shapiro, is cutting his hair at the time.

2 Write down the correct procedure for each scenario, and say whether you would summon medical aid for each case.

The information you need to record in the accident book includes:

- the date
- what happened
- where it happened
- who saw it happen
- what action was taken
- whether a doctor or ambulance was called.

Portfolio Activity

Photocopy a blank page from your salon's accident book. If you cannot do this, mock up a copy of the page using the same column headings.

Assume that all the events in the last activity took place on Monday of this week. Make the necessary entries in the accident book.

RIDDOR Regulations 1995

All workplaces, including hairdressing salons, are subject to legislation, and we will be looking at this in more detail below (see page 52). One piece of legislation is known as RIDDOR – Reporting of Injuries, Diseases and Dangerous Occurrences Regulations 1995.

Under these regulations, all work-related accidents, diseases and dangerous occurrences have to be reported.

This is a legal requirement, and the information gathered helps the authorities to identify risks, to investigate serious accidents, and to help and advise employers on any action that they should take to reduce injury, ill health or accidental loss.

The events listed on pages 46–47 must be reported.

Deaths

If there is an accident in the workplace and an employee or other person working on site is killed or suffers a major injury, or if a member of the public is killed or taken to hospital, the authorities must be notified immediately, either by telephone or via the website (www.riddor.gov.uk).

Major injuries

The following injuries come into this category:

- Fractures (other than to fingers, thumbs or toes).
- Dislocation of shoulder, hip, knee or spine.
- Loss of sight (temporary or permanent).
- Chemical or hot metal burns to the eye, or penetrating injuries to the eyes.
- Electric shock or electrical burn leading to unconsciousness or requiring hospital admission for more than 24 hours.
- Unconsciousness caused by asphyxia or exposure to harmful substance or biological agent.
- Acute illness requiring medical treatment, or loss of consciousness arising from absorption of any substance by inhalation, ingestion, or through the skin.
- Acute illness requiring medical treatment which may have resulted from exposure to a biological agent, toxins or infected material.

Over three-day injury

This is an injury which does not qualify as 'major' but which results in the injured person being away from work or being unable to carry out their full range of duties for longer than three days.

Diseases

Work-related reportable diseases include:

- some types of poisoning
- occupational dermatitis, skin cancer, chrome ulcer, oil folliculitis or acne
- occupational asthma, farmers' lung, pneumoconiosis and asbestosis infections such as hepatitis, tuberculosis, legionellosis and tetanus
- occupational cancer, certain musculoskeletal disorders and hand-arm vibration syndrome.

Dangerous occurrences

Sometimes things happen which may not result in a reportable injury but which might easily have done. Examples of this include:

- explosion of a vessel or associated pipework
- electrical short circuit or overload causing fire or explosion
- unintentional explosion or injury caused by explosion
- collapse or partial collapse of a scaffold
- explosion or fire causing interruption to normal work for more than 24 hours.

Gas incidents

Death, injury or major incident caused by piped gas or bottled gas must be reported.

Consider this

You might feel, quite rightly, that a lot of these situations are unlikely to affect you in a hairdressing salon. However, you might be surprised, when you start to think about it, at how many of them could affect you.

Make a list of the ways in which RIDDOR could relate to a hairdressing salon and then compare it with the one below. You may have thought of some others.

- A stylist is badly injured or killed by electrocution (remember, electricity and water in combination can be lethal).
- A workman fixing the lights falls off his ladder and is injured or a stylist falls off a chair or ladder on which she is standing to reach a shelf.
- Somebody falls over and breaks their arm or dislocates a shoulder, knee or hip.
- A stylist gets bleach in her own eyes or in a client's eyes.
- The receptionist is attacked whilst taking the day's cash to the bank.
- Gas fumes escape from faulty boilers.
- A stylist is diagnosed with occupational dermatitis.
- The ceiling collapses during the night because of a flood from the flat above.

The table below gives some examples of the types of incident that must be reported.

Incident	Comments
A death at work	Must be reported within ten days, no matter what the cause of death
An accident at work	Accidents have to be reported if a hospital or doctor's visit is required, or if the victim is away from work for more than three days following the accident
Employee has a work-related disease	Examples of this could be occupational dermatitis, hepatitis, asthma caused by a product used at work, or by the environment in the salon
Attack on a member of staff by another person	If the attack takes place in the workplace, it must be reported. This applies if the attacker is another member of staff, a client or a visitor
Any dangerous incident, even if nobody was injured	If your central heating boiler exploded but nobody was hurt, the matter must still be reported
A hairdresser working away from the salon has an accident or injures a client	If you spend your day off providing hairdressing to residents in a local care home, you must report any injuries or accidents to the manager of the home and to the environmental health officer

Keeping records

A record must be kept of all reportable injuries, diseases or dangerous occurrences. This must include the date and method of reporting, the date, time and place of the incident, a brief description of what happened, and the names of witnesses.

Consider this

Find out where the records of reportable injuries and dangerous occurrences are kept in your salon. You may find that there have never been any reportable incidents because they are, by their very nature, unusual. However, your manager should be able to tell you where such matters would be recorded if they did arise.

Support and maintain health, safety and security at work

You will hear a lot about 'hazards' and 'risks', so we should start by making sure that you understand the difference between the two things.

> **Hazard:** Anything which has the potential to cause harm.
>
> Risk: The likelihood of that happening, or the 'chance' (high or low) that somebody could be harmed by the hazard.

For example, electricity is a hazard. The risk of somebody being harmed by electricity might be high (if flexes are frayed, for example, or if somebody is turning on switches with wet hands) or it can be relatively low (if care is taken, and if all electrical appliances are checked according to regulations).

Risk assessment

A risk assessment is nothing more than a careful examination of what could cause harm to people within your workplace.

By carrying out a risk assessment, you can weigh up whether you have taken enough precautions or whether you need to do more in order to prevent harm. The aim is to make sure that nobody gets hurt or becomes ill because accidents and illnesses can ruin lives and can affect your business by increasing the insurance costs. You are legally required to assess the risks in your salon.

First, you need to discover whether the hazard is significant, and whether you have taken enough precautions to ensure that the risk is small.

There are five steps to follow when carrying out a risk assessment.

1   Look for the hazards.
2   Decide who might be harmed and how.
3   Decide whether existing precautions are adequate or if you need to introduce more.
4   Record your findings.
5   Review the assessment, and revise it, if necessary.

Look for the hazards

Walk around your workplace and look at what could cause harm. Ask your salon owner and colleagues what they think; they might notice things that you miss.

Decide who might be harmed and how

Don't forget new staff, young workers, clients, visitors, cleaners, colleagues and anybody else who shares your workplace.

Decide whether existing precautions are adequate

Consider how likely each hazard is to cause harm. This will help you to determine whether more should be done to prevent or reduce the risk. Each hazard needs to be rated high, medium or low.

First, ask yourself if you have done all that you can, and all that the law requires. Your real aim is to make all risks small by ensuring that you do all you can to make your workplace safe. If you find that you need to draw up an action list, give priority to the risks that are high and that could affect the most people.

Record your findings

If your salon has fewer than five employees, you do not have to write anything down, although it is useful to keep a written record of what you have done.

If there are more than five employees, the findings must be recorded. You must show that a proper check was made and how you dealt with significant hazards. You also need to show that you have taken account of the number of people involved and that any remaining risk is low.

The written record should be kept because you will then be able to show what precautions you have taken. It will also remind you to keep an eye on the hazards and precautions.

Review your assessment, and revise, if necessary

From time to time, your salon will get new equipment which may lead to new hazards. Your risk assessment therefore needs to be kept up to date. Don't think that it is just a 'once-and-for-all job'.

Take a look at the following completed risk assessment form, which might help you to prepare your own assessment.

Risk assessment for	Assessment undertaken	Assessment review
Company name: Topsy Turvy Address: Never Neverland, Somewhere over the Rainbow, PO9 7XP	Date: 11.11.05 Signed: Little Miss Perfect	Date: 11.4.06
STEP 1	STEP 2	STEP 3
List the significant hazards here: Slipping, tripping (hair cuttings, trailing wires, etc.) Fire (flammable substances) Chemicals Electrical equipment (faulty, or if staff are untrained in use) Fumes (from chemicals) Sharps Spillages	List groups of people at risk from the identified hazards: Staff and inexperienced staff Colleagues Clients Cleaners	List existing controls (or state where information can be found on risks that are not adequately controlled, and action needed). Comply with recognised industry standards. Ensure that all staff are properly trained to use equipment. Is any further action needed to control the risk?

Cleanliness

A straightforward way to reduce hazards in the salon is by making sure that the salon is kept clean and tidy at all times.

This means that all hair should be swept up as soon as the stylist has finished the cut. Hair left on the floor can be extremely slippery, and the last thing you want is a stylist slipping over with a pair of scissors in their hand.

Spillages of shampoo, conditioners, water, etc. must obviously be cleared up immediately.

If a client leaves her bag next to her chair so that people are in danger of tripping over it, ask her quietly and politely if she can move it. If it is anything other than a handbag, offer to stow it away for her until she is ready to leave.

Make sure that all unoccupied chairs are tucked under the workstation and watch out for trailing flexes from hairdryers, tongs, etc.

Replace light bulbs as soon as they fail so that the salon is always bright and well lit.

If you see something dangerous that you cannot fix yourself, report it to your manager as soon as you can. If it is something really dangerous, such as a frayed flex on a piece of equipment, remove the equipment if possible, or at least make sure that nobody uses it.

These simple precautions can reduce the potential dangers to clients and staff.

Don't think that it is somebody else's job! If you are not busy with a client, make it your business to tidy up discreetly. Keeping the salon safe is just as important as sending your clients out with a super hairdo.

Security

You need to think about security as well as health and safety. As a junior stylist, you may not be responsible for locking up the salon each evening, but you should still be aware of the regular end-of-day routine in the salon.

First of all, is there a regular end-of-day routine? It is better if there is. If you always follow the same procedure, there is less likelihood of something being forgotten. Although everybody in the salon will have some 'closing down' jobs to do, somebody will have to take the final responsibility.

Consider this

Think about your salon. Make a list of the jobs that need to be done before you can all go home in the evening.

Now compare your list with the one below. Has everything been covered?

- Sweep up hair, clean mirrors and ensure that the salon is clean.
- Turn off and unplug equipment.
- Ensure that all taps are turned off.
- Empty bins.
- Cash up and place cash in the safe or take to the night safe.
- Close and lock windows.
- Set the answering machine, if appropriate.
- Set the burglar alarm.
- Lock doors on leaving and check that they are secure.

Cash security

A hairdressing salon takes a lot of money during the course of a day and there may not be any one person who is responsible for it. If your salon has a full-time receptionist who always takes the cash, she will obviously take responsibility. However, in some salons, the stylists are responsible for charging their clients, and in those cases, it may not be so easy to keep control of the cash.

Most salons deal with this by having a system of vouchers that the stylists complete, showing the services they have provided for each client, and the amount that has been charged. At the end of the day, the manager will total these vouchers and check to ensure that the money in the till matches the total. The manager will also compare the vouchers with the appointments listed in the book to check that there is a voucher for each client. If it appears that cash is missing, the manager may decide to take control of cash handling in future.

Key Skills Activity Communication C2.1a

This activity will give you key skills evidence for communication. Discuss the following scenario with your group.

In your salon, there is a small pot for each stylist on the reception desk into which clients put tips. One day you notice that Mrs Jones puts a two-pound coin in your pot but when you empty it that evening, it does not contain any two-pound coins. You mention this to another stylist and she says that she has noticed that she is receiving less money in tips than she used to. You are worried that somebody has been stealing the tips. What could you do to ensure that it did not happen again? Who would you tell?

Regulations, regulations, regulations

Hairdressing salons, in common with all other workplaces, are subject to a number of legal regulations. These include the following.
- The Health and Safety at Work Act 1974
- Control of Substances Hazardous to Health Regulations 2003 (COSHH)
- Electricity at Work Regulations 1989
- Personal Protective Equipment at Work Regulations 1992
- Employer's Liability (Compulsory Insurance) Act 1969
- Data Protection Act 1998
- Manual Handling Operations Regulations 1992

It looks a daunting list, but nobody expects you to learn the Acts by heart. However, it is important that you are aware of the requirements and obligations contained in them, and that you know where to go to get further information.

Your salon should display a large poster entitled 'Health and Safety Law'. This is for your benefit and you should make sure that you have read it.

Portfolio Activity

Where is the Health and Safety Law poster displayed at your workplace?

What is the name of the person responsible for health and safety matters within your workplace?

The Health and Safety at Work Act 1974

Your employer has a responsibility to ensure that:

- the workplace is safe and without risk to health
- plant and equipment provided is safe to use and safe systems of working are set up and followed
- articles and substances are moved and stored safely
- exits from the workplace are kept clear
- employees receive adequate health and safety training
- adequate welfare and first aid facilities are provided
- if there are more than five employees, a health and safety risk assessment is carried out, and any measures identified are put in place
- if there are more than five employees, a health and safety policy statement is drawn up and made available to employees
- if premises are shared with another employer, co-operation takes place between employers.

As an employee, you also have responsibilities. You must ensure that:

- you take responsibility for your own actions and do nothing that could harm yourself or other people
- you co-operate with your employer and obey all health and safety instructions
- you use equipment correctly and in line with the instructions you have been given
- you do not damage or misuse any equipment that has been provided to safeguard your health and safety.

Control of Substances Hazardous to Health Regulations 2003 (COSHH)

Your employer has an obligation to control your exposure to hazardous substances in the workplace. In the salon, you will be dealing with a number of substances and chemicals and whilst most of these are safe under normal conditions, they may be dangerous if they are not used properly. Your employer should have assessed the risks posed by all substances to which you may be exposed, and should have given you appropriate training.

As part of this assessment, your employer should have completed a COSHH sheet for each product. The sheet will contain details of the contents of the

Quick tip

Taking responsibility for your own actions means thinking about consequences. For example, if you are asked to use an unfamiliar piece of equipment, on which you have not been trained, ask for help. Nobody will think you are silly if you admit that you do not know how to use something. They will think you are rather more than silly if you do not ask and cause an accident.

Dust

Toxic

Flammable

Irritant

Corrosive

Oxidising agent

COSHH symbols showing types of hazardous substances

Tips

SHUD – store, handle, use and dispose of in accordance with salon policies, manufacturer's instruction and local byelaws.

Manufacturers **have** to supply COSHH data sheets for all their products. Get one for each product.

Remember that a reaction can happen if the client is using products at home that may not mix well with salon preparations, e.g. home hair colourants.

Clients may be more susceptible to reactions if they are taking long-term medication, such as HRT or the contraceptive pill. This must be included on the client record card.

Invest in all the leaflets and latest information regarding COSHH from your local Health and Safety Executive office. **Keep up to date and keep safe.**

Remember these COSHH tips

substance, action to be taken in the event of misuse, and precautions to be taken. Each substance must also be allocated a hazard rating.

You may find one or more COSHH symbols on a product.

Remember, it is not only hairdressing products that could be dangerous within a salon. Cleaning products or bleach can also cause problems if they are mishandled. Anything in an aerosol could explode if exposed to direct heat, and it can be dangerous to breathe in the fumes from aerosol cans.

Electricity at Work Regulations 1989

These are wide-ranging regulations that apply to the use of electricity in all workplaces. As far as hairdressing salons are concerned, the regulations state that PAT testing (Portable Appliance Testing) must be carried out at regular intervals. PAT checks must be carried out by a competent person, which may be an electrician or somebody who has taken an approved PAT course.

A label will be affixed to each piece of equipment when it has been tested and a record will be kept in a special electrical safety log book.

If the tester finds that the equipment is faulty, it must be removed from use immediately and not used again until it has been repaired and re-tested. A record of the fault will be listed in the electrical safety log book, and the result of the re-test will also be entered.

Personal Protective Equipment at Work Regulations 1992

Your employer must provide you with suitable protective clothing for you to use when you are carrying out certain tasks. For example, you will be given a protective apron and gloves to use when you are colouring or bleaching hair. It is up to you to ensure that you use this protection.

Just as you have the right to insist that you are supplied with protective equipment, your employer has the right to insist that you use it. If you fail to do so, and have (or cause) an accident, you could be in serious trouble and your right to compensation could be affected.

Portfolio Activity

1 Where are the COSHH sheets kept in your salon?

2 Who has access to the sheets?

3 Find the COSHH sheets for the following and put a copy in your portfolio:

   a Hairspray

   b Washing-up liquid

   c Toilet cleaner.

Consider this

Imagine the following scenario. You are colouring a client's hair, and you do not use the protective apron and gloves that your boss insists on. You have not used this particular colour before but you are obviously allergic to it because, as soon as it gets onto your hands, your hands itch and become very sore.

You drop the bowl and splash your skirt, tights and shoes. The bowl, with the remainder of its contents, lands on your customer's very expensive new leather handbag.

What could happen? You might need to have some time off work while your hands recover. Your boss could well argue that you brought the incident on yourself by failing to wear the equipment supplied. He might therefore decide not to pay you during your absence and he will almost certainly refuse to compensate you for your ruined clothes.

Although the salon's insurance policy could be expected to cover the client's handbag, your boss will not be very pleased with you if the premium rises because of the claim.

You could also be disciplined under your company's disciplinary policy and procedures, for failing to act in accordance with

Quick tip

Remember, wearing protective clothing and using protective equipment is not an optional extra – it is essential.

Employer's Liability (Compulsory Insurance) Act 1969

All employers must have employer's liability insurance. This is to cover them against compensation claims by employees for injury or disease caused during their employment. The absolute minimum for this is £2 million but nowadays most employers choose a higher limit.

Portfolio Activity

Your employer should have their Employer's Liability Insurance Certificate displayed in the workplace.

Where is it posted?

What is the limit of cover?

£2 million seems a huge amount of money but just think of the size of a potential claim.

Consider this

Imagine the following situation. A stylist is in the stock room collecting some colour for her next client. As she reaches up for the bottle, the upper shelves, which contain files and paperwork going back several years, collapse and the stylist is trapped underneath a mass of shelving, heavy files and hair products. An ambulance is called and paramedics discover that the stylist has no feeling in her body below the neck. Further tests in hospital reveal that her back is broken. As a result of the accident, the stylist is paralysed and cannot work again. She has two young children and she is responsible for their upbringing.

How much compensation would be appropriate in this case? It is hard to put a figure on it but it would need to be big enough to support the stylist, possibly for the rest of her life, along with her two children. Child-care costs would also be incurred if the mother could no longer look after the children herself. Now, £2 million does not seem so high any more, does it?

Quick tip

A number of fraudulent companies send out reminders about data protection compliance and request a fee for entering companies on a register. These registers are meaningless and are certainly not a legal requirement. If you are in any doubt about demands for payment for data protection registration, contact the Data Protection Registrar at the following address:
Springfield House, Water Lane, Wilmslow, SK9 5AX.

Data Protection Act 1998

All businesses that have computer or paper-based records to hold personal details about their staff or clients need to register with the Data Protection Registrar. The name of the business will be placed on a public register, and the company will be required to comply with a code of practice. Under this code, the company will be required to keep information secure, and to ensure that it is accurate and is used only for the purpose for which it is collected. The company is also required to provide individuals with details of any information held on them.

Manual Handling Operations Regulations 1992

These regulations relate to the problems that can be caused by incorrect lifting and handling. You may think that they apply only to heavy industry or warehouse personnel, but you need to give just as much thought to lifting a heavy box of product in the salon as someone who works in a warehouse would to lifting a box in the depot.

Health and Safety Know How

1 Your salon must have a written Health and Safety Policy Statement which must be distributed to all employees if there are more than:
   a 10 employees
   b 12 employees
   c 5 employees
   d 3 employees.

2 In the event of a fire, the receptionist must take with her:
   a the money from the till
   b the appointment and visitors' books
   c her handbag
   d the clients' coats.

3 A risk assessment should be carried out:
   a before the salon opens each day
   b at regular intervals and when new equipment is introduced
   c when there is nothing else to do
   d after an accident has happened.

4 Your employer must have the Employer's Liability Insurance Certificate:
   a locked in the filing cabinet
   b displayed in the salon
   c in his solicitor's office
   d he does not need a certificate.

5 You should wear protective equipment:
   a when doing potentially dirty or dangerous jobs
   b as prescribed by your employer
   c when you are cleaning the salon
   d when riding your bike home.

6 RIDDOR applies to:
   a all workplaces
   b hairdressing salons only
   c only those workplaces that subscribe to it
   d hospitals and doctors' surgeries only.

Kelly's Problem Page

Dear Kelly

I am thinking of going into business on my own as a mobile hairdresser. I have just moved to a small village in a new area of the country so I could not be accused of 'poaching' my old clients. The last hairdresser in this village retired last year and the shop was closed. I cannot afford to open a shop but I think a mobile hairdresser would be very popular. I already have a list of potential clients. Are there any legal regulations that I should bear in mind?

Kelly replies:

Good for you! Yes, there are some points that you should remember. You will need insurance cover just in case anything goes wrong. With no employer to fall back on, you would be personally liable for any claims. Any reputable insurance broker will advise on this.

You may need additional insurance cover for your car, as you will be using it for business use. Again, ask your broker or insurance company.

Also, tell the Inland Revenue that you are becoming self-employed. They will tell you what you need to provide in the way of accounts and tax returns and will also advise on self-employed National Insurance contributions.

Make sure that you cost your services properly. Don't forget to take into account your travelling time. Act professionally and provide potential clients with a price list.

Remember to keep receipts for product that you buy, and for car expenses, stationery, etc. You will need these when completing your tax return.

Finally, don't be tempted to tell any fibs to the Inland Revenue about your income – the penalties are very severe when you are caught.

Kelly's Problem Page

Dear Kelly

I'm in trouble with my boss. He found out that I skipped college last week and he's really angry. It was only health and safety so it's not as if I've missed anything important, but what can I do to placate my boss?

Kelly replies:

Oh, well, as long as it was only *health and safety*! What does it matter if your clients are electrocuted or if you harm yourself inhaling fumes, or if somebody falls over something left on the floor and breaks their leg? Why should you care about regulations designed to protect you and your clients?

As you will have gathered, I'm on your boss's side. I think that the best thing you can do is read through the health and safety section of this book and make sure that you understand it. Then go and apologise to your boss (and your tutor) and tell them that you do recognise the importance of health and safety in the workplace.

More importantly, make sure that you always bear health and safety in mind when you are working in the salon.

Kelly's Problem Page

Dear Kelly

I was given a new hairdryer for my birthday, but my boss won't let me use it in the salon because she said it hasn't been PAT tested. What does this mean? It's a new dryer so there can't be anything wrong with it.

Kelly replies:

Portable Appliance Testing (PAT) needs to be done for all portable equipment used in a workplace. This basically means everything that has a plug on it.

Your boss is quite right. Every item of equipment has to be tested on a regular basis and must carry a sticker showing the date on which the last test was carried out.

The cost per item is fairly small but, of course, it all adds up when you think how many pieces of equipment there are in a salon. If you really want to use your own dryer, you could take it to your local electrical shop and they will probably be able to test it for you, or at least recommend somebody else who could.

Personally, I would keep my new dryer to use at home, and use the ones provided in the salon for work use.

Your Notes

Your Notes

UNIT7

CONTRIBUTE TO THE EFFECTIVE RUNNING OF THE SALON

Introduction

This unit consists of one practical assignment and one written paper.

The practical assignment for this unit consists of three tasks. You are required to:

- collect and analyse data relating to the productivity of your salon
- assist in stock control
- organise and monitor the work of junior members of staff in the salon.

The framework you are working towards will determine whether the written paper is to be marked externally or internally.

To meet the criteria, you will use the skills that you have developed during your Level 3 work. The emphasis is to prove your skills within a responsible position in your salon.

To complete the practical assignment correctly, you need to ensure that you are aware of the criteria against which you will be assessed.

Support effective productivity within the salon

What do you think is meant by productivity? In this context we mean improving the way resources within the salon are used so that profitability is improved.

What resources are available within the hairdressing salon?

Perhaps the most important resource is the human resource, i.e. the staff of the salon. Other resources include product, equipment and, one you might have overlooked, time.

A few minutes' thought will show you that whoever has control of the appointments book in the salon is in control of two important resources – personnel and time.

Arranging appointments so that the stylist has time to provide a good service to each client, without wasting time between clients, is quite an art, but it is essential that it is mastered.

In order to run an efficient appointments book, you need to know how long to allow for each type of service (cut, blow dry, perm, highlights, colour, etc.). If more than one stylist will be working with the same client, you will need to make sure that each stylist is available at the appropriate time, so the client does not have to wait too long. This situation is quite likely to arise if your salon has some stylists who specialise in colouring, and others who specialist in cutting.

You can see therefore that it is very important to make sure that each stylist's time is used effectively, since this can dramatically increase staff productivity within the salon.

Portfolio Activity

How long is allocated in your salon for each of the following services?
- Shampoo and blow dry (short hair)
- Shampoo and set (short hair)
- Shampoo, set and putting long hair up
- Semi-permanent colour
- Highlights, including cut and blow dry
- Consultation before first treatment
- Perm

Friday 18th November 2005

Time	Senior Stylist Tamara	Senior Stylist Miles	Senior Stylist Sioban	Stylist Natasha	Junior Stylist Guy	Stylist Ebony
9.00 am			Farley			Stirling
9.15 am	Zena	Rawlings	Full			Wedding
9.30 am	Cut	Consultation	Head	Payne		Consultation
9.45 am	Finish		Foils	Gents		
10.00 am		King	xxxxxxxxxxxxxxxxxx	Cut	Goslind	Dridge
10.15 am	Piddicombe	Root			Root	Full
10.30 am	Cut	Retouch		McDonald	Retouch	Head
10.45 am	Perm		Farley	Skin test		Foils
11.00 am	xxxxxxxxxxxxxxxxxx		Finish		Minn	xxxxxxxxxxxxxxxx
11.15 am	xxxxxxxxxxxxxxxxxx	King	xxxxxxxxxxxxxxxxxx	Goslind	Semi	xxxxxxxxxxxxxxxx
11.30 am	xxxxxxxxxxxxxxxxxx	Cut		Cut		
11.45 am	Piddicombe	Finish	Bradley	Finish		Dridge
12.00 pm	Cut	LUNCH	Treatment	Minn	xxxxxxxxxxxxxxx	Cut
12.15 pm	Finish	LUNCH	xxxxxxxxxxxxxxxxxx	Scrunch	Cleaning	Finish
12.30 pm		LUNCH	Cut	Dry	xxxxxxxxxxxxxxx	
12.45 pm		LUNCH	Finish		xxxxxxxxxxxxxxx	
1.00 pm	LUNCH	Crowley	LUNCH	LUNCH	LUNCH	LUNCH
1.15 pm	LUNCH	Cut	LUNCH	LUNCH	LUNCH	LUNCH
1.30 pm	LUNCH	Perm	LUNCH	LUNCH	LUNCH	LUNCH
1.45 pm	LUNCH	xxxxxxxxxxxxxxxxxx	LUNCH	LUNCH	LUNCH	LUNCH
2.00 pm		xxxxxxxxxxxxxxxxxx		Chloe		
2.15 pm	Wallis	xxxxxxxxxxxxxxxxxx	Green	Treatment	Reed	Collis
2.30 pm	Treatment	Crowley	Wet		Semi	Skin test
2.45 pm		Cut	Cut	Chloe		
3.00 pm	Wallis	S/S		Hair		Reed
3.15 pm	Cut			Up	Jones	Cut
3.30 pm	Restyle		Lock	xxxxxxxxxxxxxxxx	Treatment	Finish
3.45 pm	Finish	Crowley	Root			McQueen
4.00 pm		Comb out	Retouch			Cap
4.15 pm	Savage			Jones	Smithe	H/L
4.30 pm	Cut	Steine	Lock	Cut	Skin test	
4.45 pm	Finish	Gents cut	Finish	Finish		McQueen
5.00 pm						Finish

An appointments book

Portfolio Activity

Look at the appointments book above. It should be clear to you that the time could be better used. Draw up a sheet of your own and rebook the appointments to make better use of the stylists' time.

Another way to improve the use of resources is to increase the amount of product sold. You will remember that in Unit 1 we looked at ways in which you could offer clients the opportunity of buying suitable products.

You will only improve the productivity of the retail sales operation within the salon if your clients make repeat purchases. This means that it is essential that your clients are offered good advice, and sold products that suit their hair and which will produce the effect they want.

Key Skills Activity Application of Number (N2.1, 2.3) and Communication (C2.1a, 2. 3)

You should be familiar by now with the criteria for Communication key skills. This practical task offers excellent opportunities for you to meet some of these criteria. After each task we have listed the key skills criteria that it could cover.

Note: The most important people in any business are the clients so, if you want to know how to improve your business, they are the people to ask.

Your first practical task is to ask clients their opinion of the services you provide and ask them for ideas about the services they would like you to offer.

You should present your findings to your manager, along with suggestions of changes that could be made to improve the service you offer, both in terms of hairdressing services and sale of retail products.

Your task, therefore, is to:

1 Carry out a survey of at least 30 clients, and collate and present the findings in an appropriate manner. (N2.1.1, 2.1.2, 2.1.3)

As part of this, you will need to design a questionnaire that gives you the information you require. So, the first thing to do is to sit down and think about what information you need. There is no point in collecting data just for the sake of it.

You need to find out whether the clients were satisfied with the service they received. This covers everything from the way they were greeted to their thoughts about the final look.

You also need to know what extra services or aftercare the clients would like you to provide.

Your survey should be carried out over a period of at least two weeks to make your findings more accurate.

Prepare a short report summarising the results of your survey. (N2.3, C2.3.1, 2.3.2, 2.3.3 and 2.3.4)

2 Hold discussions with the other staff in the salon to gain ideas for:

a) improving the services you offer to clients (referring to the report you have produced)

b) improving productivity

c) solving problems that arise within the salon so that all staff work together effectively, and are therefore as productive as possible. (C2.1a.1, 2.1a.2, 2.1a.3)

3 Using the results of your survey, and the discussions you have held with staff, prepare proposals for the salon manager or owner about ways in which your salon's productivity and the services it offers to the clients could be improved. (C2.3.1, 2.3.2, 2.3.3 and 2.3.4)

Note: Make sure that you discuss all this with the salon manager or owner before you start. Your manager might not appreciate you holding staff meetings and surveying the clients without his or her knowledge.

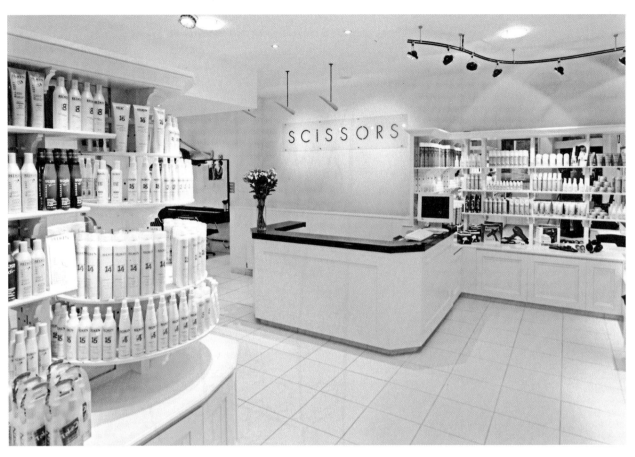

Well-stocked and attractive displays will help to increase sales

Maintain stock control procedures

It is important that regular stock checks are carried out, for several reasons:

- to ensure that you do not run out of product
- because stock is vulnerable to theft
- so that out-of-date or damaged product can be removed from the shelves.

Consider this

Which method of stock control does your salon use? Do you have a stock card for each item or do you use a computerised system? How often do you carry out stock checks? Who is responsible for ordering new stock?

A standard method of stock control is to use stock cards for each item. Each item has a minimum and maximum quantity allocated to it, and the idea is that your stock is never higher than the maximum level and never lower than the minimum level. When you carry out your stock check, you should order enough product to bring your stock control levels up to the maximum stock level. Bearing this in mind, carry out the activity overleaf.

It is important to carry out regular stock control checks

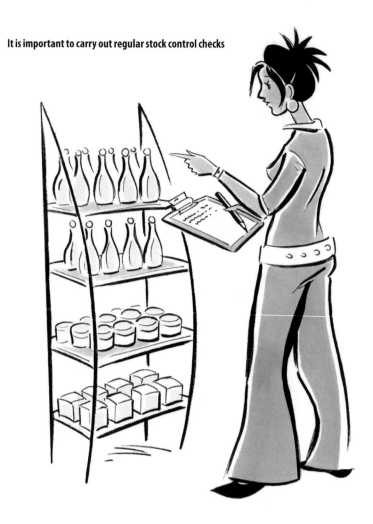

Portfolio Activity

A selection of your stock control sheets show the following information:

Product	Maximum Stock	Minimum Stock
Hair spray	30 cans	5 cans
Shampoo – dry hair	10 bottles	3 bottles
Shampoo – greasy hair	10 bottles	3 bottles
Conditioner – dry hair	5 bottles	2 bottles
Styling wax	4 jars	2 jars
Leave-in tonic	3 bottles	1 bottle
Replacement blades	4	1
Paddle brushes	2	1

When you carry out a stock check, you find that you have the following in stock:

10 cans of hair spray, 8 bottles of shampoo for dry hair, 4 bottles of shampoo for greasy hair, 3 bottles of conditioner for dry hair, 4 jars of styling wax, 1 bottle of leave-in tonic, 3 replacement blades and 2 paddle brushes.

Write an order to your supplier for the new stock that you need.

When stock is delivered, you should carry out the following checks.

- Check the delivery note against the order to ensure that they both match.
- Check the stock delivered against the delivery note, to ensure that the items that have been delivered are those listed on the note.
- Check that all items are in good condition.
- If any items are damaged or missing, you should follow your salon's procedures.

Portfolio Activity

Using whichever system is already in place in your salon, your task is to:

a) carry out a stock check, and complete the appropriate documentation fully and accurately

b) identify any damaged or out-of-date items, and separate these from other stock items. Deal with these in the way prescribed by your salon and make a note about what action you took.

Having carried out your stock check some products will have to be reordered.

Contribute to planning, organising and evaluating work

As you progress through your hairdressing career, you will take on increasing responsibility for other members of staff, especially younger staff who are undergoing training.

The amount of involvement that you have will depend on the salon in which you work, but in order to gain your qualification, you will have to show that you have done some work in this area. The key skills activity overleaf asks you to allocate work to junior colleagues.

Key Skills Activity Communication C2.1a, C2.3

The following task will not be formally assessed, but it will enable you to prove that you have covered the criteria for this part of the unit. It can also be used to provide evidence for Communication key skills.

1. Draw up a list of tasks that could be carried out by junior colleagues. (C2.3.1, C2.3.2, C2.3.3)

2. Draw up a list of junior colleagues and make a note of the level of guidance that each requires. (C2.3.1, C2.3.2, C2.3.3, C2.3.4)

3. Consult your manager about the work activities that you have identified and check whether these meet the salon's current requirements.

4. Ensure that your junior colleagues are informed about the work activities that have been allocated to them. (C2.1a.1, 2.1a.2 and 2.1a.3)

5. Make a record of any verbal instructions that you give. (All criteria within C2.3)

6. Encourage your colleagues to ask questions if they are unsure about the responsibilities and activities that have been allocated to them. (C2.1a.1, 2 and 3)

7. Evaluate the work performance of your junior colleagues.

8. Complete any feedback paperwork that is used in your salon.

9. Give constructive feedback to your colleagues about their work performance. (C2.1a.1, 2 and 3)

10. Make sure that all your communications with your junior colleagues are conducted in such a way that goodwill, trust and confidentiality are maintained.

11. Make a record of all these activities, without breaching confidentiality and with the consent of all parties involved. (All criteria within C2.3)

Contribute to the Effective Running of the Salon Know How

1 Stock checks should be carried out:
   a regularly, at least once a week
   b when things start to run out
   c when the rep calls
   d they are not necessary.

2 The one resource that cannot be replaced is:
   a stock
   b staff
   c time
   d the building.

3 A client asks for an appointment with a stylist who is already fully booked. Do you:
   a put her name down anyway – the stylist will have to manage
   b apologise and offer an alternative appointment
   c suggest she goes to another salon
   d tell her she should have booked earlier.

4 You are fully booked and one of your clients turns up 20 minutes late. What would you do?
   a Send the client away and tell her she is too late.
   b Start her service as soon as she arrives and make the rest of your clients wait.
   c Explain to the client that you will fit her in as soon as you can, but give her the opportunity to transfer to a stylist who has a free appointment.
   d Explain that you will have to charge extra for the inconvenience.

5 A client wants to buy a bottle of shampoo but you have run out of the type she needs. Would you:
   a suggest she goes to the chemist next door and tell her that the shampoo they sell is just as good
   b sell her the nearest thing you have
   c tell her that you will get some from the supplier as soon as possible and offer to ring her when it arrives
   d tell her you have sold out?

6 When stock is delivered, you should check the stock against the delivery note to ensure that:
   a you are being charged the right price
   b what has been delivered is what is on the delivery note
   c what has been delivered is what you ordered
   d none of the stock is damaged.

Kelly's Problem Page

Dear Kelly

When my boss was on holiday, a new sales rep called. He was really nice and told me about some good special offers that his company had available. I put in an order for quite a lot of stock, as it's always a good idea to stock up when prices are low, but when my boss came back, he told me off. He said that I should not have ordered anything without carrying out a stock check first, and he was also annoyed because I had ordered product that we had never used before.

He phoned the company and asked them to take the stock back. I was so embarrassed that I hid in the staff room when the rep came back.

I am really fed up with being treated like a junior with no responsibility.

Kelly replies:

Well, you haven't proved that you can handle responsibility, have you? Stock checks are important because stock costs money and no business wants its money tied up in stock sitting on a shelf. The idea is to keep enough product so that you do not run out, but not too much more.

It might be a good idea to stock up when prices are low if the stock is likely to be used fairly quickly, but not if it is just going to sit on a shelf. Also, you ordered product that your salon does not generally use. You should not have done this without the agreement of your boss. When you are trying new product, you should buy small quantities to start with, not large quantities just because it seems cheap.

I have a suspicion that you got carried away because the rep was 'really nice'. That isn't terribly professional or responsible.

Kelly's Problem Page

Dear Kelly

Our salon does not have a receptionist, and whoever is free has to answer the phone. When I have to make appointments, I always leave plenty of time so that the stylist does not have to rush and the client does not have to wait.

One of the stylists keeps telling me off, because she says that I should fit in more clients, and not leave so much time between appointments. So I started to fit more clients into her column, and now she says that she's not superwoman and that she can't cope with all the clients I've given her.

How on earth can I cope with somebody so unreasonable?

Kelly replies:

There is a happy medium which you don't seem to have reached yet. You need to speak to the stylist and your manager and make a list of how long each activity should take – e.g. how long for a cut, how long should you allow for a shampoo, how long for a blow dry? Once you have this list, you will be able to allocate the stylists' time more accurately.

When you are making appointments, always ask the stylist if you are not sure whether she can fit in the client's service.

You are quite right to want to give the stylist enough time to carry out the service properly, and you are also right to realise that clients will not want to wait for too long. However, time is money and it is important that the stylists' time is used as productively as possible.

Your Notes

Your Notes

Your Notes

SECTION 2

PRACTICAL SKILLS

UNIT2

PROVIDE HAIR AND SCALP TREATMENT SERVICES

Introduction

This unit consists of one practical assignment and one internal written paper. The practical unit consists of two tasks – one to provide hair and scalp protective treatment services and one to provide hair and scalp corrective services.

To meet the criteria, you will use the skills that you have developed during your Level 2 work, specifically in unit numbers 202 (old standards) or H9 (new standards).

To complete the practical assignment correctly, you need to ensure that you are aware of the criteria against which you will be assessed. You must also make sure that you have the correct equipment available within the salon to complete the tasks.

Provide hair and scalp treatment services

Special treatments

As part of your consultation with the client, you will need to find out if any special treatments are required. You will find it helpful to use the recommended consultation sheet (on pages 198–199) to record the consultation.

Treatments may be required to *protect* certain hair types, or to *correct* the effects of harsh treatments or non-infectious scalp conditions.

Protective treatments may be needed for conditions such as:
- dry hair, possibly as a result of the effects of mild physical or chemical damage
- dry, flaky scalp
- split ends
- dry, brittle hair.

If you use a protective treatment before carrying out chemical processes, the porosity of the hair will be evened out. This will help to improve the condition of the hair and ensure that the chemical process gives better results.

Corrective treatments may be needed to deal with:
- more severe effects of physical or chemical damage
- severe, non-infectious, scalp conditions.

If you use a corrective treatment before direct heat is applied, the damage to the hair cuticle will be minimised.

During your consultation with the client, it is important that you discuss not only the treatments that are required, but also the causes of the condition for which treatment is needed. There are two main reasons for this:

- Your client will feel involved in the consultation.
- Your client will be better able to look after her hair between visits so that further damage is avoided.

The table opposite identifies some possible causes of damage to hair.

Cause	Comments
External factors: • brushing, combing, backdressing • shampooing • blow drying and styling • hot rolling and brushing • crimping and tonging • wearing pastiche, dreadlocks, etc.	You need to examine the hair carefully in order to check its condition. LOOK at the hair closely FEEL the surface of the hair EXAMINE the skin of the scalp TALK to your client ASK if she has any hair problems LISTEN to what is said If a simple treatment such as shampooing is carried out incorrectly, it will be reflected in the condition of the hair. If necessary, advise your client on the best way to treat her hair at home.
Weather: • sun, wind, sand, sea and salt • extremes of climate – hot, cold, dry, humid • moisture	Hair needs to be protected from the effects of the weather. For example, most people nowadays are aware of the potential effects of sun on the skin, and take care to use an appropriate sun cream. It is also important to recognise the effects of sun on the hair, and to cover up with a sun hat. During your consultation, you could ask your client if she is about to go on holiday, and offer advice before the damage is done.
Chemicals: • hairdressing processes including perming, colouring and bleaching • swimming in the sea or in pools, if salt or chlorine is not rinsed out of the hair thoroughly afterwards	The damage caused by over-application or wrong use of chemicals may be made worse by other factors, such as the weather. It is important, therefore, that you address all the possible causes of damage when discussing the matter with the client.
General health and lifestyle: • good health is reflected in the hair and skin. A balanced diet, with plenty of fresh foods, contributes to good health • disease, and the drugs used in the treatment of diseases, may affect the hair and skin • genetic factors may affect hair growth, texture and strength • pregnancy and childbirth – although the hair of pregnant women is usually at its best, stress and tiredness following the birth can cause a deterioration • women often report increased hair loss after childbirth. This is because fewer hairs are shed during pregnancy, with a 'catch up' following the birth	You may be able to gain information about a client's health or lifestyle during the consultation. You will probably recognise changes in a regular client, and you need to discuss these without being intrusive. It is important to recognise that the effects of poor health may not be apparent in the hair until some time afterwards. You should reassure your client that these effects can be cleared up. A positive approach is always best.

Possible causes of damage to hair

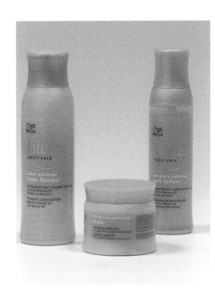

Conditioning products can add moisture or nutrients to the hair

Selecting suitable products

After your client consultation, you will need to select a suitable product to use on the client's hair.

You will have gone to a lot of trouble to ensure that you have chosen the right product. However, a product will only work to its full advantage if it is applied properly, so make sure that you read the instructions.

You must check:
- the length of time required for the process
- the equipment needed
- the method of application.

As well as reading instructions, get into the habit of noting the ingredients in each product that you use. You will find that similar ingredients are used by most manufacturers. The table below gives examples of some ingredients used in shampoos.

Shampoo	Hair/scalp type	Benefits
Jojoba oil	Dry	Adds moisture
Coconut oil	Dry	Adds moisture
Almond oil	Dry	Adds moisture
Lanolin	Dry	Adds moisture
Soya	Normal	Cleanses
Strawberry	Normal	Cleanses
Lemon	Greasy	Removes grease
Egg and lemon	Greasy with sensitive scalp	Removes grease
Medicated	Dandruff	Relieves condition
Coal tar	Psoriasis	Releases scales and relieves condition
Zinc	Dry scalp	Relieves itchiness
pH balanced	Damaged/coloured hair	Returns hair to normal pH
Soapless	All types	Used before chemical processes
Beer	Fine/limp	Adds body

There are two main types of conditioner. Both types penetrate, to help repair the chemical structure of fibres within the cortex.

Protein conditioners and treatments – These will add nutrients to the hair, to help rebuild from within. In some cases this may thicken the hair. These conditioners also help to smooth the surface of the hair and close the cuticles to protect against further damage. They also help strengthen the hair shaft.

Moisture-based conditioner and treatments – These will add moisture to dehydrated hair to rehydrate, smooth and repair the hair shaft. They can also be used to help minor scalp problems.

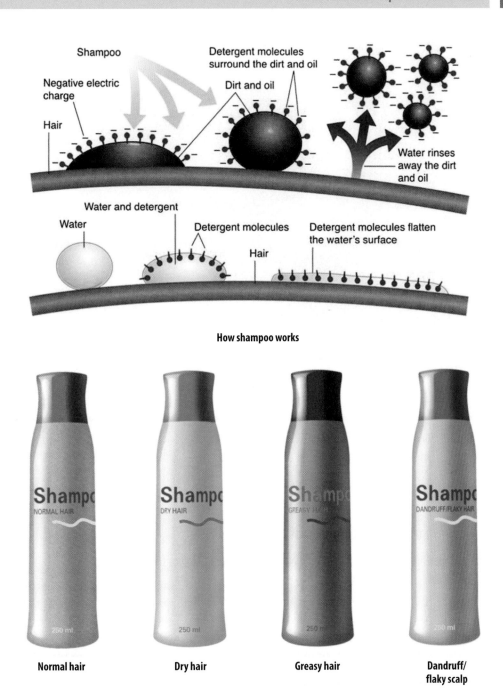

How shampoo works

| Normal hair | Dry hair | Greasy hair | Dandruff/ flaky scalp |

Different shampoos will be suitable for different clients

Having selected your product, make sure that you apply it correctly following the manufacturer's instructions. Is it applied directly from the bottle, or with the aid of a bowl and brush?

A backwash basin is more comfortable for most clients when their hair is washed

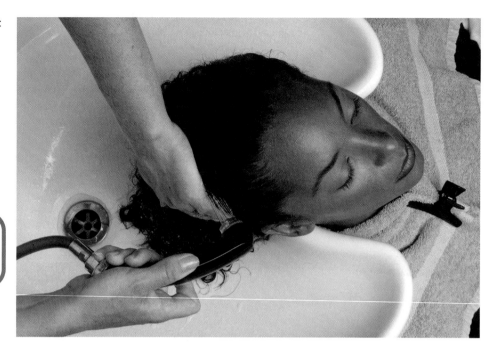

Quick tip

When listing ingredients, don't be fooled by the exotic-sounding aqua — it just means water!

Consider this

Look at the products your salon uses for each of the following hair types.

- Dry.
- Normal.
- Greasy.

Select a shampoo and conditioner that you would recommend for each type, and list the ingredients.

Visit a supermarket or chemist, and look at a shampoo and conditioner recommended for each of these hair types. Make a note of the ingredients.

How do the ingredients in the retail products differ from those in the professional salon products?

Would the salon products be better? Why do you think so? Remember, you may have to explain this to a client one day.

Portfolio Activity

The products that your salon stocks are more expensive than some brands that are sold in chemists and supermarkets, but you are convinced that your products are best.

Write a short (one A4 page) handout that can be left on your reception desk, explaining why your products are worth buying. Concentrate on shampoos and select one for each hair type.

Remember, you must *not* take this as an opportunity to be rude about other products — you should just point out the advantages of using yours, with reference to the ingredients used and the benefits they offer.

Massage

During the conditioning treatment, you will massage the scalp. There are several reasons for this. How many can you think of?

Massage:

- *manipulates* the skin and muscles. It is usually carried out with the hands, but the use of vibro-massage or high-frequency machines can enhance the effects
- *improves* the *blood flow* to the skin
- helps *improve muscle tone* and *soothes nerve endings*
- aids in the process of *removing waste products* from the skin surface
- *increases the flow of nutrients* via the blood supply.

There are several hand massage movements, some of which are shown in the spider diagram below.

Quick tip

A good massage will help relax and prepare your client for the following services.

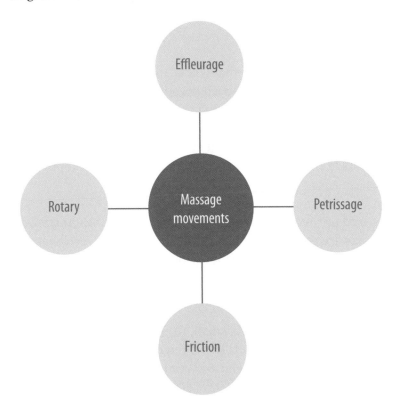

Some of the most commonly used hand massage movements

Effleurage

Effleurage is a smoothing, stroking action applied to the scalp with firm but gentle movements of the hands and fingertips in a slow rhythmic manner. It is used at the beginning and at the end of each massage treatment to relax muscles and ease tension.

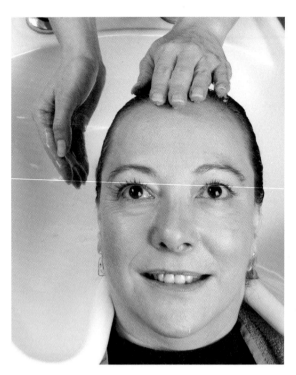

Effleurage movement

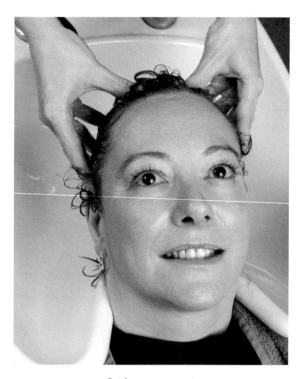

Petrissage movement

Petrissage

Petrissage is the main movement that will be used during the conditioning process. Petrissage is a slow, firm, deep kneading movement in which the skin is gripped by the pads of the fingers and rotated over the skull. It increases blood circulation and gives deeper stimulation to the muscles and glands. It will help to break down adhesions/fatty congestions, assist in the elimination of waste products and increase the flow of nutrients/blood supply.

Friction

Friction is used during shampooing. Friction is also a kneading movement and the fingers are rotated in opposite directions. Unlike petrissage, the movements are very fast and vigorous with the fingers moving over the surface of the skin.

Rotary

Rotary massage consists of quick, small, firm, circular movements used when shampooing, using the pads of the fingers to clean the scalp. It will help to remove dirt and grease, and will stimulate the scalp ready for the more gentle massage which is to follow during conditioning.

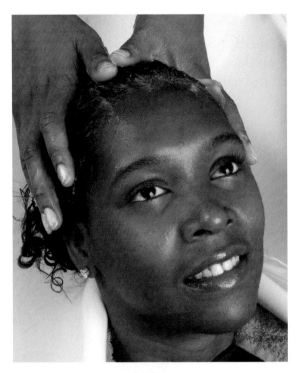

Friction

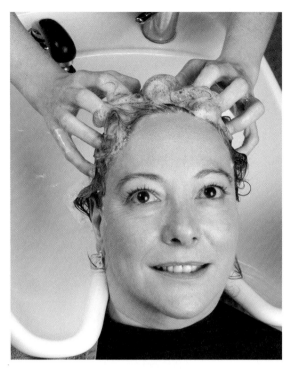

Rotary massage

Heat treatments

Once you have applied your treatment, you can select an appropriate method of heat to develop the treatment.

Equipment used for processing treatments includes:
- steamer
- accelerator
- roller balls
- radiant heat/infra-red lamps
- scalp massage electrical equipment
- vibro-massager
- high-frequency unit.

Steamer
Steamers produce moist heat through the evaporation of distilled water. Steam will flow around the hair, which will allow the hair to expand and soften. This enables the treatment to penetrate into the cortex to produce the maximum benefit from the product.

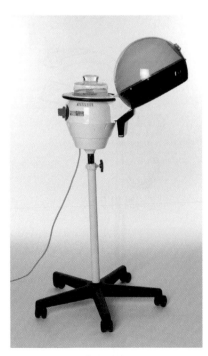

A steamer

Climazone

Climazones, or accelerators, produce dry heat. Like steamers, they help the deep penetration of conditioning products. The use of this equipment will help the treatment to be absorbed and reduce processing time.

Roller ball

A roller ball is similar to a climazone but uses infra-red heat and has a fan. The source of heat moves continually to ensure that the whole head is covered. The roller ball can be used during other hairdressing services.

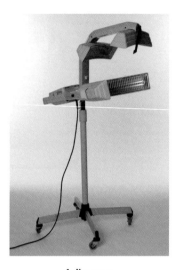

A climazone

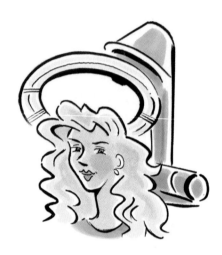

A roller ball

Heat lamp

Radiant heat and infra-red lamps are similar to climazones in that they irradiate heat to the head and the hair.

Vibro-massager

A vibro-massager is an electrically operated massager designed to produce vibratory movements similar to the petrissage and friction hand movements.

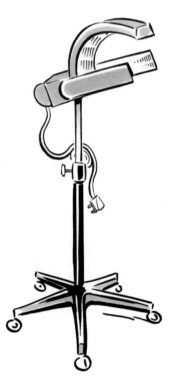

A heat lamp

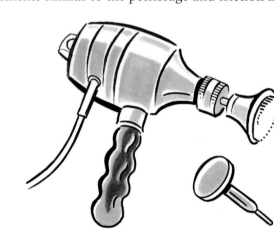

A vibro-massager

High-frequency unit

A high-frequency unit is a portable generator which produces a high-voltage and low-voltage current strength. It produces an electrical current, either directly or indirectly.

Direct method – With the direct method, glass electrodes are applied to the skin through either a round, glass bulb (for use on the bare areas of the face or scalp in a rotary action) or a glass comb/rake (for use on the hair of the head, passing through the hair upwards towards the crown).

Indirect method – In the indirect method your client would hold a metal bar or saturator in her hands. When the current is switched on, it is directed onto the scalp by your hands. As your fingers touch the client's skin, the electrical current flows from the machine to the client through the bar that she is holding and then to your fingers. You can then massage the scalp.

The current will be low for the first few treatments and will only be increased if the client can tolerate it. Treatment should not exceed 12 minutes.

You should *not* use high frequency if:
- there are signs of inflammation
- evidence of a skin disorder is present
- the client is receiving medical treatment
- the machine is damaged
- you are near water.

When using electrical equipment, you *must*:
- follow health and safety procedures
- read and follow the manufacturer's instructions
- ensure that you have had training on the piece of equipment
- follow the Electricity at Work Act guidelines
- make a visual check before using equipment
- ensure that every portable piece of equipment (i.e. any equipment that has an electric plug) carries a sticker to confirm that it has had PAT checks (i.e. Portable Appliance Testing)
- ensure that there are no frayed flexes or loose plugs and that there is no evidence of damage to any machine.

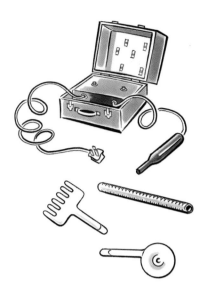

A high-frequency unit

Quick tip

If in doubt, do not use the machine.

When you have completed the processing, make sure that the product is thoroughly removed. Towel dry the hair, removing all excess water, then comb the hair to remove any tangles.

You should complete the record card now, if you have not already done so.

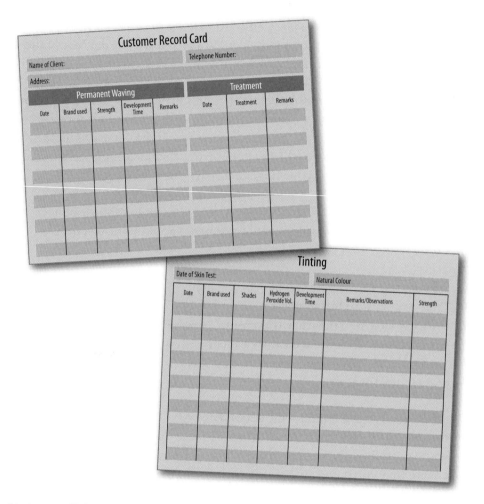

A record card must be filled in neatly

Hair condition

As a hairdresser, you will realise that the condition of the hair can have a disproportionate effect on a person's well-being. How many times have you heard comments like these?

- This new hairstyle makes me feel like a million dollars.
- As long as my hair looks OK, I feel great.
- My hair is in a terrible state, and I feel dreadful.
- I've just got over flu, I feel depressed, I've got spots and my hair is driving me mad.

Your job is to ensure that the client leaves the salon looking her best, and with a positive plan of steps to take to keep her hair in good condition.

Key Skills Activity Communication C2.1a

This group discussion could provide evidence for Communication key skills. Try to arrange for a tutor or assessor to observe the discussion, and to assess you on C2.1a.1–3.

Group discussion:

Split into groups of three or four and discuss the following scenario with other members of the group.

Imagine that you are undertaking a consultation with a client. She has been to the salon before, but not for several months. Last time you saw her she was pregnant. Now the condition of her hair isn't very good. The ends are split, the style has grown out, and the hair is dry and looks lifeless.

During the consultation, your client tells you that she has a two-month-old baby. Then, to your horror, she bursts into tears and says that she is tired, she gets no sleep, and her hair is driving her mad. She is losing hair every time she brushes it and she is frightened that she will lose all her hair.

1 What action would you take?

2 What advice would you give the client?

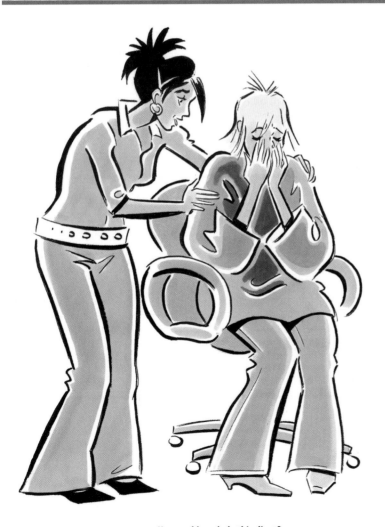

How could you help this client?

I hope that the first thing you would do is to reassure the client that nearly everybody has trouble with their hair following childbirth.

Your client would probably appreciate a cup of tea or coffee – with a small baby, she probably doesn't get waited on very often. You should then discuss the effects of pregnancy on the hair and the after-effects of childbirth, including tiredness and stress. You should explain why new mothers lose hair following the birth and reassure her that this will not lead to baldness.

Quick tip

You should have the pleasure of seeing your client leave the salon looking good, feeling spoilt and feeling confident.

You should discuss an appropriate style and suitable aftercare. A mother with a new baby will need a style that is easily managed, and that will look good if it is simply washed and blow dried. We are talking about a good cut, a simple and easily managed style, and suitable conditioning treatments in the salon.

More serious conditions

In the last section (page 81), we looked at the damage that might be caused to hair by various factors. From time to time, you may find a client suffering from a more serious condition, which will call for different action from you.

The following chart (on pages 93–95) shows the types of condition that you might come across, and identifies the symptoms and causes, as well as suggesting possibly remedies.

Portfolio Activity

When you read through the following chart, you realise that many of the junior members of staff in your salon will not have encountered some of the conditions listed – after all, you do not see clients with these conditions every day. Your juniors may be the first people in the salon to take a close look at a client's hair, when they are shampooing (especially if looking after existing clients, who may not need a consultation at every visit).

You realise that it is unrealistic to expect your juniors to be able to recognise all these conditions straight away, so you decide to prepare some checklists for them. Each checklist will deal with three of the conditions. Your juniors will be given one checklist each week.

Prepare the first week's checklist, choosing the three most commonly met conditions, and explaining what the staff should look for, what action they should take if they find the condition, and the treatment that will be recommended.

Make the checklists clear and easy to understand, and make sure that the facts are correct.

	Condition	Symptoms	Causes	Remedy
Bacterial infections				
	Barber's itch (sycosis barbae)	Small, red or yellow spots around follicle; inflammation and irritation; burning sensation. Usually found in beard area	Bacterial infection	Medical treatment required
	Folliculitis	Small yellow spots with hair in middle	Bacterial infection	Medical treatment necessary
	Impetigo	Weeping blisters with dry yellow crust	Bacterial infection	Medical treatment essential. Highly contagious
Infestations				
	Head lice (pediculosis capitis)	White specks attached to hair shaft, near scalp. Check behind ears and at nape of neck. Itchy and contagious. Common in children	Parasites that lay eggs, which stick to hair. Spread by head-to-head contact or by sharing brushes, etc. Multiply rapidly	Treatment may be purchased from pharmacist. Highly contagious. Any tools that have been used on somebody with head lice must be sterilised before being used again
	Scabies	Irritating red spots and lines on skin	Parasites	Highly contagious. Medical treatment essential

	Condition	Symptoms	Causes	Remedy
Non-infectious conditions				
	Male pattern baldness	Thinning hair, baldness, receding hairline	Hereditary	None as yet, although medical treatment is being investigated
	Monilethrix	Beaded hair	Uneven production of keratin. Usually hereditary	Gentle treatment
	Psoriasis	Thick dry scales, raised. Usually silver in colour, and found behind ears	Stress or anxiety. Overproduction of epidermal cells. May be hereditary	Coal tar shampoo. Medical treatment from doctor
	Pityriasis capitis (dandruff)	Small grey or white scales on hair and scalp. May itch	Stress or anxiety. Overproduction of epidermal cells, which are subsequently shed	Specialist shampoo with ingredients such as selenium sulphide or zinc pyrithone. Conditioning creams and serums may be applied directly to scalp
	Sebaceous cyst	Lump on scalp	Blockage in sebaceous gland	Surgical removal or draining. May burst if treated harshly, so care must be taken in salon
	Seborrhoea (greasiness)	Excessive oil on scalp	Stress or anxiety. Overactive sebaceous gland	Spirit lotions. Specialist shampoo for greasy hair

	Condition	Symptoms	Causes	Remedy
	Trichorrhexis nodosa	Hair broken off; hair rough and swollen along shaft	Physical damage or harsh treatments	Restructuring. Cutting and reconditioning hair
	Warts	Small, raised lumps of skin	Viral infection. Spread by touch or direct contact	Not contagious unless damaged, so treat carefully in salon
	Alopecia areata	Bald patches	Stress, shock, severe anxiety	High-frequency treatment. Medical treatment from doctor
	Fragilitis crinium (split ends)	Hair ends dry and split, or rough	Chemical treatments. Harsh rubbing with towels, overheating	Split ends cut off. Hair reconditioned

Fungal infection

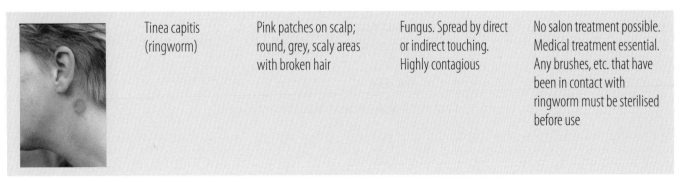

	Condition	Symptoms	Causes	Remedy
	Tinea capitis (ringworm)	Pink patches on scalp; round, grey, scaly areas with broken hair	Fungus. Spread by direct or indirect touching. Highly contagious	No salon treatment possible. Medical treatment essential. Any brushes, etc. that have been in contact with ringworm must be sterilised before use

Shampooing/conditioning Know How

1 In order of priority, treatments are used to:
a protect the hair
b nourish the hair
c add shine to the hair
d correct excessive damage.

2 Hot water taps should be turned off during the massage process in order to:
a increase humidity
b conserve hot water
c clean the basin
d reduce the processing time.

3 Heat should be added when processing a treatment to:
a keep the client more comfortable
b allow the treatment to penetrate
c speed the processing time
d warrant the extra charge.

4 What is meant by the term emulsify?
a to lather the hair
b to clean the hair
c mixing shampoo and water
d rinsing the hair

5 Physical damage to the hair may result from:
a shampooing
b sunlight
c combing
d sleeping.

6 The process which may cause most damage to the cuticle is:
a straightening
b shampooing
c perming
d bleaching.

7 Hair in good condition usually has a pH value of:
a 3–4
b 6.5–7.5
c 10–12
d 4.5–5.5.

8 Hair elasticity refers to the hair's ability to:

a   be treated

b   break

c   stretch

d   stretch and return.

9 Which of the following ingredients in shampoo is used for dry hair?

a   strawberry

b   zinc

c   coconut

d   beer

10 Which of the following conditions requires medical treatment?

a   fragilitis crinium

b   monilethrix

c   pityriasis capitas

d   psoriasis

Kelly's Problem Page

Dear Kelly

The shampoo and conditioner that we sell in the salon are quite expensive, compared to the ones you can buy in the supermarket. Our manageress keeps telling us to promote these products to our clients, but I find it hard to explain why they should spend £7.99 on a bottle of shampoo instead of £2.50.

Do you think salon products are a rip-off?

Kelly replies:

No, I don't think they are a rip-off, but if you think they are, your clients will probably get the same idea.

Look at the ingredients in the salon products and compare them to those in branded products. In my experience, you use less of a salon product so a bottle lasts much longer. Also, your clients can be sure that a product that has been recommended by you will suit their hair types. Your salon may have a policy of allowing clients to return products with which they are not happy – very few supermarkets would make a refund on a half-used bottle of shampoo.

You should make positive recommendations to your clients, but remember that it is unprofessional to be rude and critical about other manufacturers' products. If your client simply cannot afford £7.99 for a bottle of shampoo, be ready to give her advice about a suitable product that could be purchased from a chemist. If you have any special offers on your products, make sure that your client is aware of them. Some manufacturers offer sample sizes, which can be purchased relatively cheaply.

Kelly's Problem Page

Dear Kelly

A client came into the salon last week and when I started to shampoo her hair I found that she had head lice. I called out to another stylist to come and have a look. I told the client to go away and come back when she had got rid of the head lice. I also told her that she should make sure she washes her hair properly in future because people with clean hair don't get head lice.

I said that we couldn't dry her hair as the head lice would be blown all over the salon. She was very angry and asked to speak to the manager. I told her that the manager wasn't in but that he would have told her the same as I had. She rang the manager later that day to complain about me. I feel that I handled a delicate situation very well but my manager was angry. What do you think? After all, it wasn't my fault she had head lice.

Kelly replies:

Well, there's one client you won't see again. Firstly, head lice are not a result of having dirty hair. Normal shampoos are ineffective in removing them. Having discovered the head lice, you embarrassed your client by calling out to another stylist. You should have spoken to the client quietly and confidentially, and reassured her that most people get head lice at some time in their lives.

You should have recommended that she visit the chemist to buy a product to deal with the problem and reassured her that you would fix another appointment as soon as the problem had been dealt with. The head lice would not have been blown all over the place by a hairdryer, and you should not have sent her away with wet hair. You should have cleaned all equipment you used discreetly after the client had left the salon.

You sent her away feeling dirty, embarrassed and ashamed and with no advice about how to deal with her problem. Not only are you unlikely to see her again, but I doubt whether many of her friends will come to you either. Your boss is right to be angry with you.

Your Notes

Your Notes

Your Notes

UNIT3

CUT HAIR TO CREATE A VARIETY OF FASHION LOOKS

Introduction

This unit consists of one practical assignment, one written assignment and one written paper.

The practical assignment for this unit consists of three cutting tasks. You have to create fashion looks on one man, one woman and one child. These are the recommended clients but others may be substituted provided they cover the range of cutting techniques and effects. During these cuts, you are required to carry out a range of cutting techniques.

The written assignment will require you to have sufficient knowledge of how to cut a client's hair with varying requirements using a variety of cutting techniques to achieve fashion looks. You will need to understand the importance of taking into consideration factors that may influence the outcome of the haircut.

The framework that you are working towards will determine whether the written paper is to be marked externally or internally.

To meet the criteria, you will use the skills that you have developed during your Level 2 work, specifically in unit numbers 204 (old standards) or H6 (new standards).

To complete the practical assignment correctly, you need to ensure that you are aware of the criteria against which you will be assessed. You must also make sure that you have the correct tools and equipment available within the salon to complete the tasks.

Cut hair using a variety of techniques

Women's hair

Client 1 – Your client wants a short layered look. She requires texturising to give a broken-up look rather than a smooth one. You are to thin and taper the hair and she likes a razored effect.

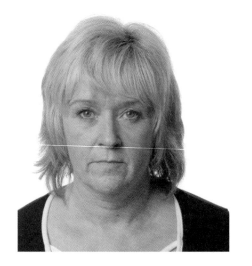 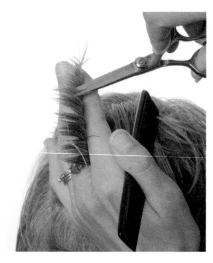 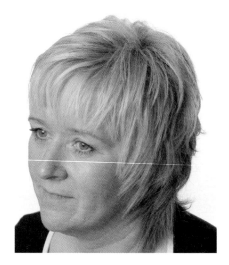

| Before | During | After |

Men's hair

Client 2 – Your client wishes to have a fashion look which is short and graduated and cut close around the nape and the ears.

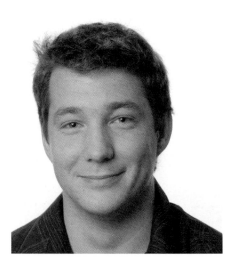 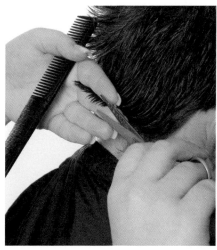 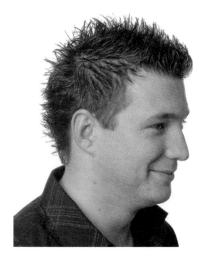

| Before | During | After |

Children's hair

Client 3 – Your client's parent wants her to have a one-length look that rests above the collar line. The parent tells you that the child does not like the feel of a razor or clippers.

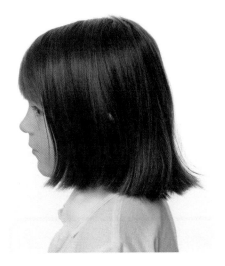

Before

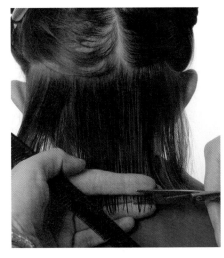

During

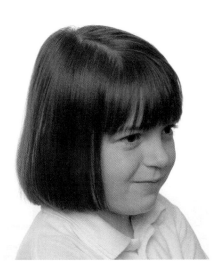

After

Textured look

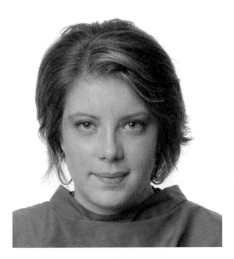

Client before cut – consultation has been carried out with the use of visual aids/pictures to establish the desired style

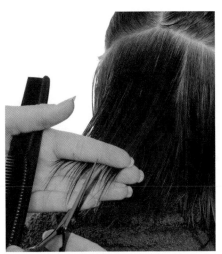

Tools used included scissors to chip into and blunt cut, and the razor to help remove bulk in order to achieve and create a textured, choppy look

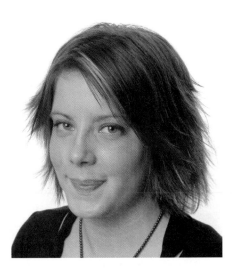

The completed look enhances the broken, textured fashion look that was required. Finishing products were used according to hair type and texture

Evidence collection

When carrying out your assignments, you or a colleague should (with the client's permission) take photographs before, during and after the service. You can then arrange your photographs and add short explanations of what each picture represents. This will become part of your evidence and can also be used for part of the written assignment.

When using visual aids and style books, etc, include any pictures that you have selected along with your consultation sheet. This will not only provide you with extra evidence, but it will help you to create a picture story of the service you have provided.

Don't forget – all this evidence will help you to achieve a higher grade.

Health and safety

Portfolio Activity

Listed below are some health and safety incidents that you should be aware of when cutting. For each situation, say why it is dangerous, and what you should do to minimise the danger:

1   incorrect alignment of clipper blades
2   exposed sharps
3   putting sharps in your pocket
4   stylist wearing open-toed shoes
5   hair not swept up
6   broken teeth in comb
7   client has hay fever
8   loose wires on clippers
9   unsterilised tools
10 empty first aid box.

Let's see how your answers compare with ours.

1   Incorrect alignment of clipper blades – the client may be cut.
2   Exposed sharps – these are particularly dangerous if there are children about, as they could be cut if they pick them up.
3   Putting sharps in your pocket – think what could happen if you bend over. You could cut yourself through your clothing.
4   Stylist wearing open-toed shoes – she could get hair splinters in the feet, or stab them if sharps are dropped.
5   Hair left on floor – this is amazingly slippery, and could cause a fall.
6   Broken teeth in comb – would pull the hair and possibly graze the scalp.
7   Client with hay fever – if the client sneezes suddenly she could be cut.
8   Loose wire on clippers – could cause an electric shock.

Quick tip

It might sound obvious, but scissors and razors are sharp. When cutting, make sure that you abide by all the health and safety regulations that have been put in place to protect you, your colleagues and your clients.

9 Unsterilised tools – could be responsible for passing on infection/infestation and does not look professional.

10 Empty first aid box – if an accident did happen, you would not even be able to provide a plaster.

Key Skills Activity Communication C2.1b, 2.3

You can use the information from the last task to provide key skills evidence, and you can also cross-reference this to Unit 8 (Health and Safety).

1 Prepare a talk on 'Health and Safety' in the Salon that you can give to new staff who are just beginning their hairdressing training. Use the above information as a guide to the sort of things you can include, but you should be able to think of others too. Your talk should last for 4–5 minutes. Use the rest of your group as your audience and present your talk.

This will give you evidence for Communication C2.1b.

Make sure that you:

- speak clearly in a way that suits the subject, purpose and situation (2.1b.1)
- keep to the subject, and structure your talk to help listeners follow what you are saying (2.1b.2)
- use appropriate ways to support your main points. (2.1b.3)

2 Prepare a handout (at least 500 words long) summarising the main points of your talk, which your audience can take away with them to remind them of the things they need to be aware of. Also, prepare a notice that you can display in the staff room of your salon, reminding staff of the importance of health and safety in the salon.

This will give you evidence for C2.3.

Make sure that you:

- present relevant information in a format that suits your purpose (2.3.1)
- use a structure and style of writing to suit your purpose (2.3.2)
- spell, punctuate and use grammar correctly (2.3.3)
- make your meaning clear. (2.3.4)

Before the cut

Remember to carry out the consultation procedures that we looked at in earlier units. Use your consultation sheet, and make sure that you gather information on:

- the client's face shape
- contraindications
- hair texture
- hair type
- hair length
- hair condition
- hair volume and movement
- hair growth patterns

- the client's age, lifestyle and body shape
- the reason for the visit to the salon – a special occasion, maybe?

Face shapes

To complete this unit, you will need a more comprehensive knowledge of face shapes.

Taking account of your client's face shape is extremely important when carrying out any service, especially cutting. The overall effect of the style will depend on how well your client's face shape has been complemented. During the cutting process, you can dramatically change the shape of the style to flatter your client's face shape.

Portfolio Activity

Draw each of the following shapes onto a piece of paper.

a Square

b Rectangle

c Round

d Long

e Heart

f Oval

g Pear

From these simple shapes you can draw and create each face shape, adding dotted lines to soften each shape.

To the shapes you have created, you can now add hairstyles that you feel will flatter each face shape.

Your drawings should reflect the following:

Square face – You need to create roundness to reduce the angular jawline and forehead. Avoid square-cut bobs or long, straight styles. You need to add wispy layers around the face and height at the crown to elongate the shape. Add fringes where possible.

Rectangular face – Avoid too much length; it will lengthen the face shape even more. Avoid centre partings. Try side partings instead. Try to add fullness at the sides. A short to mid-length style with layers is good.

Round face – Avoid jawline-length styles and centre partings. You need to create fullness and height at the crown, but no width at the sides. Height at the front will also help to balance the shape. Soften the jawline by adding layers. Keep some length to help create the image of a longer and narrower face.

Oval face – This is often considered to be the perfect face shape which will suit most hair styles. The oval face shape is the illusion that we want to create with the other face shapes. Avoid covering up your perfect face shape.

Long face – This is much the same as rectangular (long has a softer, less square, jawline). Add a fringe and avoid too much length. Avoid straight, one-length hair. Add some layers to add different lengths in the style.

Face shapes

The oval face

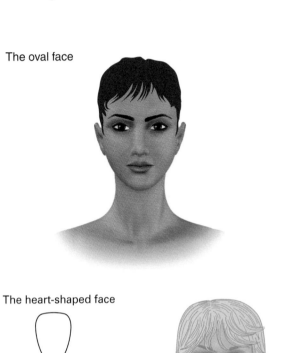

The round face

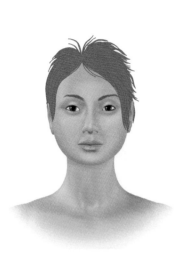

To turn into
an oval

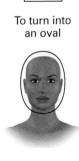

The heart-shaped face

To turn into
an oval

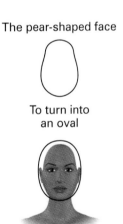

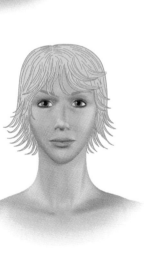

The pear-shaped face

To turn into
an oval

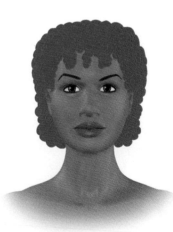

The rectangular-shaped face

To turn into
an oval

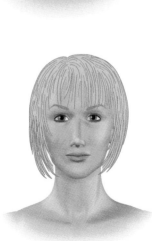

The square face

To turn into
an oval

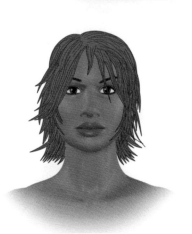

Heart-shaped face – Make the most of the nice jawline. Try chin-length styles. Add a fringe to soften the forehead. You can create a short style, but to balance the shape you will need to leave some weight in the nape area. Avoid styles that will emphasise the upper face. Avoid severe, slicked-back styles and too much height at the crown.

Pear-shaped face – Avoid very short styles and too much width around the jawline. You want to create width above the cheeks and soften the jawline. Add a fringe and soft layers.

To complete the written assignment successfully, you will need to revise the following topics.

Cutting tools

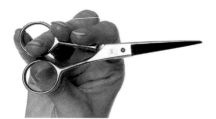

Scissors

Your selection of cutting tools is an individual choice. You will need to choose the correct tools for the specific effect that you wish to create. You must be able to control whichever cutting tool you choose, and it must be comfortable to hold. The edges must be sharp, or you can damage the hair, and the experience will also be uncomfortable for the client.

Scissors

Scissors can produce a variety of techniques. These are the most important tools for a hairdresser. They vary in size, design and price. When choosing scissors, you should try different pairs to find ones that are comfortable to hold and which suit your hands. Scissors adapt to the hands that are using them, so it is best not to let anybody else use your scissors.

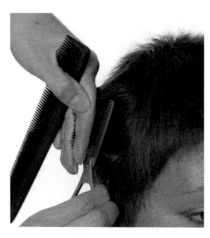

Thinning scissors

You should look after your scissors by sterilising them in an ultra-violet cabinet or autoclave or by using alcohol, sterile wipes or sprays.

Thinning scissors

These remove bulk from the hair without removing length. The aesculapian scissors have notches in the blades. The size of the notches varies and determines the amount of hair that is removed. They should be looked after in the same way as scissors. Aesculapian scissors should only be used on dry hair.

Cutting comb

You will probably also need a cutting comb. These are available in different sizes according to your needs, to suit the type of hair you are working with.

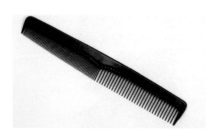

Cutting comb

Razors

These are used mainly to produce a tapered, thinned and texturised effect. The most commonly used razors are the open or cut throat razor, shapers or safety razors.

Razors have interchangeable blades. The blade must always be sharp to produce clean cuts. Razoring should always be carried out on wet hair as this reduces the friction on the hair, and is more comfortable for the client. Look after your razor in the same way as your scissors. Remember to dispose of the used blades in the yellow sharps bin.

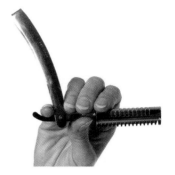

Hairdresser's razor

Clippers

Clippers are generally used for short, graduated, clubbed styles, and for tidying around the nape line and the ears. Clippers should always be used on dry hair. Although they are most commonly used in gents' styling, some ladies' styles also require the use of clippers.

Most clippers have adjustable blades to determine the fineness of cutting. With the addition of grades/clipper attachments, you can alter or vary the length of the cut.

The higher the grade of clipper you attach, the longer the hair will be. The lower the grade, the shorter the hair.

To look after your clippers, you should remove loose cuttings and then spray the blades with sterilising clipper spray. Clippers should be oiled after each use.

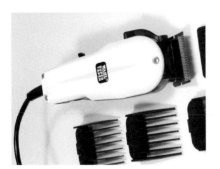

Clippers

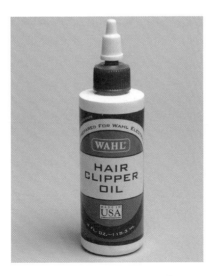

Clipper oil will help to maintain your clippers

Quick tip

Cutting tools must be handled correctly and with care. Maintain them well to prolong their life and to ensure that they give you the best possible results with each cut.

Summary of cutting techniques

Technique	Effect	Tools used	Wet or dry hair
Club cutting	Cutting straight across the mesh	Mainly scissors or clippers. Can use razor	Scissors or razor: wet or dry Clippers: dry
Scissor over comb	Cutting hair by lifting the hair up with the comb and cutting it	Scissors	Wet or dry
Clipper over comb	Cutting hair this way gives a blunt, straight edge to the ends of the hair	Clippers	Dry
Texturising	Point cutting the hair. Produces softer, broken edges	Scissors	Wet or dry
Thinning	Cutting the hair with thinning scissors will remove extreme bulk, not length	Aesculapian scissors or scissors on dry hair Razor on wet hair	Wet or dry
Razoring	Tapering to remove bulk and some length	Razor	Wet
Freehand	Cutting the hair without using hand to hold the line. Hair falls into natural shape. Good for fringes	Scissors	Wet
Graduating	Cutting the hair so that the top layers lie above the underneath layers. Low layering – very little graduation. High layering – step graduation. Top layers are shorter than the underneath layer. The effect created will depend on the degree of graduation	Scissors	Best achieved on wet hair
Layering	Cutting the hair so that the layers fall in a uniform fashion. Gives a total layered look	Scissors	Best achieved on wet hair
Tapering	Slithering movement with scissors on dry hair. Slicing movement with razor on wet hair. Removes length and bulk and encourages curl	Scissors, razor	Best achieved on wet hair

Advantages and disadvantages of cutting hair wet or dry

You will have to decide whether to cut your client's hair wet or dry. Each has some advantages and disadvantages.

Advantages	Disadvantages
Wet hair	
• More precise sectioning and lines	• Makes it difficult to discover the natural growth patterns
• Hair is easier to manage and control	
Dry hair	
• Easier to identify growth patterns	• Discomfort for client (hair flies everywhere)
• Easier to see the amount of bulk to be removed from the hair	• Harder to control and keep even tension
	• Client may have dirty hair

Portfolio Activity

For each of the following clients, state:

● any consultation information

● the chosen style and why it has been chosen

● method of cutting

● tools to be used

● aftercare advice.

You may find it helpful to collect photographs/pictures to support your descriptions.

Client 1 has shoulder-length, thick density, naturally straight hair with grown-out layers. She has a permanent colour on her hair, but it feels in fairly good condition. The client requires a modern fashion look. She would like to remove some of the bulk and introduce a fringe to her heart-shaped face.

Client 2 has short, fine, virgin hair. She is growing her hair into a classic shape, and has a round-shaped face and a double crown.

Client 3 has long, one-length, medium density, naturally wavy hair. She requires a modern style, although she would like to keep some length. She has an oval-shaped face and a slight cowlick. She would be happy with a high maintenance style.

Client 4 has mid-length, coarse, layered hair with the remains of a previous perm on the last 5 centimetres (2 inches). She requires a shorter style to remove the remainder of the perm and would like a more modern look. However, she does not want her hair cut too short at the nape. She has a long-shaped face.

Cutting Know How

1 Thinning of the hair should never be carried out:
a at the nape area
b on the fringe
c on the crown
d around the hairline.

2 Aesculapian scissors should never be used on:
a dry hair
b wet hair
c curly hair
d straight hair.

3 Which method of cutting retains the bulk?
a club cutting
b razor cutting
c taper cutting
d thinning

4 It is important that the hair is carefully assessed prior to cutting in order to:
a impress the client
b determine the condition of the hair
c determine the cutting method to be used
d determine the angle to be used.

5 Precision cutting is usually carried out on wet hair because:
a it allows the hair to fall more naturally
b wet hair is easier to cut than dry hair
c hair should only be cut wet
d dry hair cutting gives a tapered finish.

6 Which face shape is considered to be the perfect shape?
a round
b square
c long
d oval

7 What is the advantage to cutting the hair when it is dry?
a saves time
b easier to control
c easier to identify growth patterns
d more comfortable for your client

8 Prioritise the following list of health and safety risks in order of importance when carrying out any cutting service.
   a sharps in a pocket
   b stylist wearing open-toed shoes
   c unsterilised tools
   d empty first-aid box

9 How is the basic haircut cross-checked?
   a follow guidelines
   b opposite direction to sections taken during cutting
   c using hands to check balance
   d using the mirror to ensure the cut is even

10 Short graduation means:
   a the top layers are longer than the underneath layers
   b the underneath layers are shorter than the top layers
   c the hair is all the same length
   d very little graduation, as in a wedge.

Kelly's Problem Page

Dear Kelly

My manager has booked me in to do a haircut on a three-year-old next week. I am very nervous about this as I have never cut a child's hair before.

Any tips, please?

Kelly replies:

You are right to realise that there are special considerations to be taken into account when cutting a child's hair. Some children love going to the hairdresser, but others hate it.

If a child is not happy, try to find out why. It may be the cape or gown that the child dislikes; it may be the high chair that some salons use; or it may just be fear of the unknown.

If a child is very upset, you should not attempt a cut. It is a good idea if the child can be brought into the salon before the appointment for the cut, to familiarise him or her with the place and the equipment that will be used. When the appointment is made, suggest to the parent that the child brings a favourite small toy or teddy bear, so that he or she has something familiar to hold. Bribery also works with young children – a few chocolate buttons or raisins can work wonders (but make sure that you get the agreement of the parent first!).

When you start the cut, remember that children can make unexpected moves and that it would be unrealistic to expect them to sit still for a long period. Make sure that you are prepared for this.

Do not attempt a complicated cut on the first occasion. A simple trim, which finishes before the child has had time to become bored or worried, will ensure that he or she is happy to return at a later date.

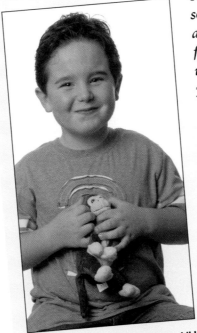

Having a special toy to hold can help a child

Kelly's Problem Page

Dear Kelly

There is one client who comes into the salon occasionally and we all dread being asked to cut her hair. She never makes an appointment, so whoever happens to be free when she comes in has to cut her hair. She is a really nice lady, but her hair is never very clean. She never wants a wet cut; she always says that she will wash her hair when she gets home. It is really unpleasant having to cut dirty hair.

We have asked our boss to refuse to book her in, but he says that we take everybody.

Any ideas?

Kelly replies:

I sympathise. It is unpleasant having to cut dirty hair, although most hairdressers have to face it at some time or another. I realise that your boss does have a business to run, but he also needs to think about his staff.

Why don't you suggest that the next time the client comes in, she is told that you are no longer doing dry cuts, because a wet cut always gives the best results. Perhaps your boss will agree that she can have a free shampoo.

After the cut, you could just give a simple blow dry so the client does not have to leave with wet hair.

Make sure that whoever does the cut that day does a really good job so that the client is persuaded that wet cuts are a good thing.

Your Notes

UNIT4

PERM HAIR TO CREATE A VARIETY OF FASHION LOOKS

Introduction

This unit consists of one practical assignment, one written assignment and one written paper.

The practical assignment for this unit consists of three perming tasks. You are required to perm two different clients' hair to create a variety of fashion looks. During perming, you are required to use a variety of techniques. This assignment can be carried out on a man or woman provided that the clients chosen cover the range of perming techniques and effects.

The written assignment will require you to have sufficient knowledge of how to perm a client's hair with varying requirements using a variety of perming techniques to achieve fashion looks and effects. You will need to understand the importance of taking into consideration factors that may influence the outcome of the perm.

The framework you are working towards will determine whether the written paper is to be marked externally or internally.

To meet the criteria, you will use the skills that you have developed during your Level 2 work, specifically in unit numbers 205a (old standards) or H12 (new standards).

To complete the practical assignment correctly, you need to ensure that you are aware of the criteria against which you will be assessed. You must also make sure that you have the correct tools, products and equipment available within the salon to complete the tasks.

Perm hair to create a variety of fashion looks

Client 1 wants a fashion look that will give either root lift or a spiral perm.

Client 2 wants a permed fashion look that will follow the direction of her preferred style.

Client 3 wants a permed fashion look that will create a varied curl effect. She would like some hair to be more loosely curled than other hair. You can carry out a weave wind or a double wind (piggyback).

When carrying out your assignments, you must select your clients carefully, and ensure that the look that you produce suits the client and her hair.

You need to make the most of any assessment opportunities, so if you have a client whose wishes fall into either of these categories, you should ask if you may use them for your assessment.

Do you remember what was said about taking photographs when we looked at the cutting assessment? The same applies to perming assessments and you should be able to build up a good portfolio containing photographic evidence.

Health and safety reminder

Perming uses strong chemicals and you must remember to:
- follow all health and safety procedures
- read and follow manufacturer's instructions
- wear appropriate personal protective equipment (PPE).

When applying perm lotion and neutraliser you must remember to do the following.

1   Wear an apron to protect your clothes from any splashes. The chemicals can discolour fabrics.
2   Protect yourself from contact dermatitis. This has caused real difficulties for some hairdressers to the point that they have had to change careers. Don't let this happen to you. Always wear gloves when applying perm neutraliser or lotion and ensure that there is no contact with the skin.
3   Remember that your client needs protection too. Use a gown, plastic cape, cotton wool, barrier cream and a neck trough, and you will minimise any dangers to the client and her clothing.

Quick tip

You should have noticed that Client 1's two wishes are completely opposite to each other. Root lift will create minimal curl, whereas a spiral perm will create tight curls.

Quick tip

Ensure that you follow these three steps as they will be an important consideration towards your grading during your assessments.

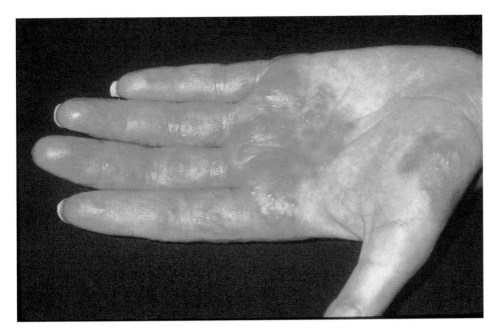

Protect your hands against contact dermatitis

Consultation

Remember the consultation procedures and the hair and scalp analysis that you need to follow before carrying out the service. Use the consultation sheet to remind yourself of the importance of the following factors.

- **Client's requirements** – These will determine the style, size of rod and the technique that you will use to achieve the effect.
- Carry out any necessary **tests** before you begin.
- **Client's face shape** – Will the chosen style suit her?
- **Contraindications** – Is the scalp free of cuts/abrasions/infections/infestations?
- **Hair texture** – This will help determine which lotion strength you should use.
- **Hair porosity** – This will determine how quickly the perm lotion is absorbed. Do you need pre-perm treatments?
- **Hair length and density** – Remember that long, heavy hair will require smaller rods, as the weight will pull on the curls.
- **Hair condition** – Carry out necessary tests to ensure that the condition is compatible with perming. If in doubt, postpone the treatment!
- **Direction and degree of movement required** – This will determine which technique to use, and the size of rod selected.
- **Growth patterns and curl patterns** – The natural movement will help determine the best direction for perming. If the hair is naturally wavy, you will need to add less curl than you would if the hair was straight.
- **Temperature** – Remember that the temperature of the salon in which you are working will have a strong influence on the development time.

Different perming techniques

There are different perming techniques which you can use to create different effects. These include piggyback (or double) winding, spiral winding, weave perming and root perming, as shown below.

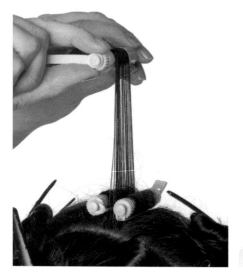
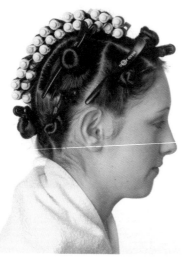
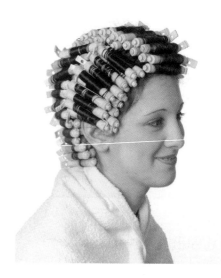

Piggyback or double winding

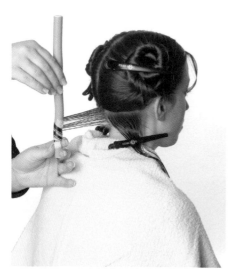
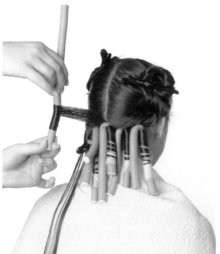
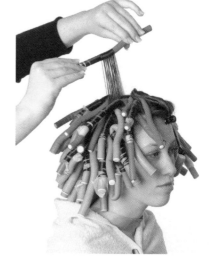

Spiral winding

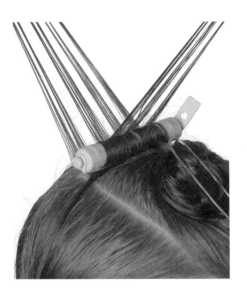
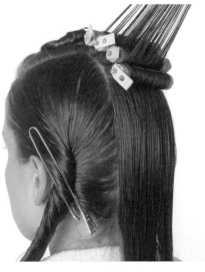
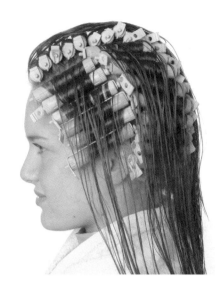

Weave perming

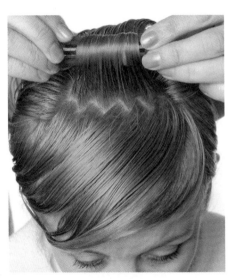
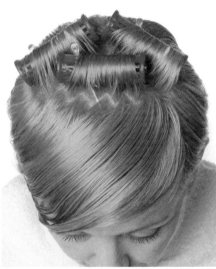
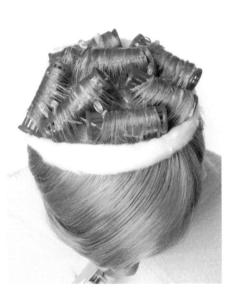

Root perming

Perming lotion and strengths

Having a perm is a major step. Provided that you have carried out your analysis correctly, you can build a picture of the desired results. Now you need to select the best product, to ensure that you create the best possible result.

There are two types of perm lotion: alkaline and acid.

Alkaline perm lotion:
- has a pH value of approximately 9.5 – the higher the pH, the more damage it will cause to the hair
- is suitable for all hair textures
- is effective on strong, coarse, resistant hair

- can be used to pre-dampen the hair
- requires no additional heat
- produces an S-shaped development test curl
- swells the cuticle and enters the cortex
- is long lasting.

Acid perm lotion:
- is kinder to the hair structure
- is suitable for fine, sensitised, porous and previously chemically-treated hair
- has an acid pH
- may require additional heat
- must be activated by mixer after reading manufacturer's instructions
- test curl divides into equal sections
- can need longer processing time
- gives a softer curl formation.

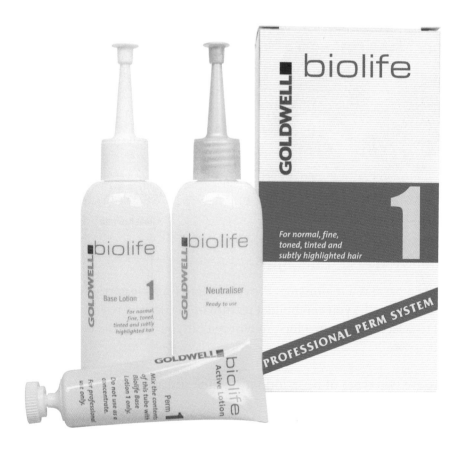

There are many different products suitable for permed styles

Consider this

Which type of perm do you think would be less damaging to the hair?

Why?

Within these two groups, there are a number of different perm strengths, all suitable for different types of hair, which includes:

- resistant/difficult to perm hair
- normal/virgin hair
- coloured hair
- dry, damaged or sensitised hair
- highlighted hair.

Portfolio Activity

Look at the stock in your salon. How many different types of perm do you stock? Can you identify one for each of the hair types shown above? Are there any others?

Perming rods

There is another choice to be made – the size of rod to use. You need to remember:

- larger rods produce larger curls or waves
- smaller rods produce tighter curls.

If you use small rods in easy-to-perm, fine hair, the hair is likely to frizz. If the rod is too large, it will not curl enough. So, this is obviously an important choice, and the best way to find out the size of rod and the amount of perm lotion that you will require is to carry out a test curl. Look at the chart on page 126 for choices of rods.

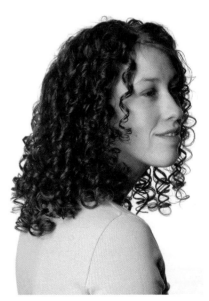

A perm can create beautiful natural-looking curls

Perming rods and their uses

Type of rod	Uses of rod
Traditional	This type of rod is the most commonly used. It is used in a variety of ways to produce many different effects
Spiral	This type of rod is used to create spiral curls on medium to longer-length hair
Wella Formers	Used to create soft waves on medium-length hair
L'Oreal Techni-wavers	Used to give volume or soft waves on shorter-lengh hair
Bendies	Used to create various effects, including spirals, curls and waves, on most hair lengths
Pin-curl clips	Used to create volume and lift on shorter hair; must be plastic as metal clips may react with chemicals used during perming

Quick tip

Remember to carry out a test curl.

- Take a test cutting and wind the hair on the chosen rod size.
- Apply lotion and develop, following the manufacturer's instructions.
- Rinse as normal and blot dry.
- Apply neutraliser and develop.
- Unwind the rod and look – is the curl enough to create the required result?

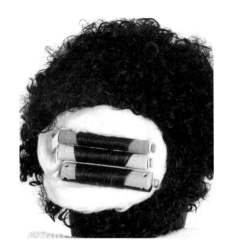

A pre-perm test curl

Portfolio Activity

For each of the following clients, state which:

- lotion type
- strength
- rod size
- technique

you would use. Don't forget, you can always say 'no' if you think that a perm would not be advisable.

Client 1 has thick, heavy, naturally dry hair, and requires a spiral wind to create a tight curly effect.

Client 2 has fine, sparse hair. She has had perms for several years, and usually leaves around three months in between. However, her last perm was not successful. She currently has no colour on her hair, but occasionally likes a semi-permanent colour. She wants body, rather than curl.

Client 3 has short, coarse, virgin hair, which has a natural wave. The wave is not sufficient for your client as she requires a wash-and-leave look.

Client 4 has medium texture, tinted hair. She is currently wearing her hair in a modern, layered look. She requires a soft curl with not too much root lift.

Client 5 has 60% head of bleach highlights. Her hair is short, thick and layered, and is in reasonable condition. She requires a medium curl and she likes to blow dry her hair every day.

Theory of perming

Warning: here comes the science bit!

Perming involves three stages.

- Stage 1 – softening
- Stage 2 – moulding
- Stage 3 – fixing

Stage 1 – softening

The perm lotion swells the cuticle, so that the perm can penetrate into the cortex. Some acid perms need additional heat to allow this to happen.

Stage 2 – moulding

The perm lotion enters the cortex where it deposits hydrogen. The hydrogen attaches itself to the disulphide bonds and breaks them apart into sulphur bonds. Not all disulphide bonds are broken during perming. The hair, which is now softened, will take on the shape of the perm rod. This is called moulding.

Stage 3 – the fixing stage

Neutralising removes hydrogen from the cortex by adding oxygen, a process called oxidisation. This process joins together the sulphur bonds to reform the disulphide bonds in their new position. This process firmly fixes the curl.

Perming involves three stages

Perm lotion opens and swells cuticle scales

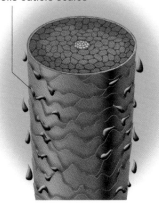

1 The softening stage

Before perming, disulphide bonds intact

The hydrogen attaches itself to the disulphide bonds and breaks them into single sulphur bonds

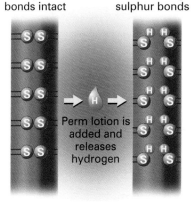

Perm lotion is added and releases hydrogen

2 The moulding stage

Neutraliser is added and oxygen is released. Oxygen joins with the hydrogen to make H_2O (water)

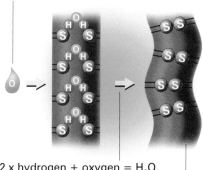

$2 \times$ hydrogen + oxygen = H_2O, which is rinsed from the hair

Sulphur bonds re-form to make disulphide bonds in a newly curled formation, which permanently fixes curl

3 The fixing stage

Portfolio Activity

A client is concerned that a perm might damage her hair and wants to know how the process works. With the aid of simple diagrams, and in your own words, describe the chemical processes at each stage of the perming process.

The diagrams you produced for the portfolio activity should look like this

Diagram of the
softening process

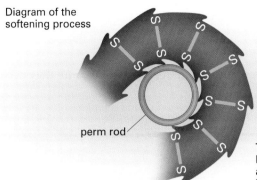

perm rod

The cuticle scales
have lifted slightly
and the disulphide
bonds are still intact

1 Softening

Diagram of the
reduction process

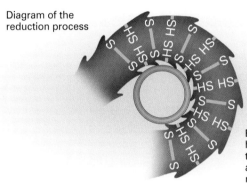

By the addition of
hydrogen, 25–30% of
the disulphide linkages
are broken during the
reduction process

2 Reduction

Diagram of the
oxidation process

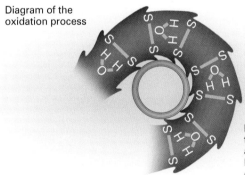

By the addition of oxygen,
the hydrogen is attracted
away, allowing the sulphur
bonds to reform into
disulphide linkages.

3 Oxidation

Key Skills Activity Communication C2.1b

You could use the portfolio activity above to provide key skills evidence. Why not give a talk to the other members of your group, describing the chemical process at each stage of the perming process?

2.1b.1 requires you to speak clearly in a way that suits your subject, purpose and situation.

2.1b.2 asks you to keep to the subject and structure your talk to help listeners follow what you are saying.

2.1b.3 specifies that you should use appropriate ways to support your main points. The diagrams you produced for your portfolio activity, either drawn onto OHP sheets, produced for a PowerPoint presentation, drawn on a flip chart, or photocopied and handed out to the audience, would meet this requirement.

Once the perm has been completed, you must update the client's record card.

Record cards

We have mentioned record cards in every unit so far as they are essential.

Portfolio Activity

What information do you think should be included on your client's record card? Make a list and then compare it with the one below.

Information needed on record card	Reason
Client's name	Self-explanatory
Telephone number	In case you need to contact your client – to alter an appointment, for example
Date of treatment	There needs to be a time lapse between certain treatments. You will also find it useful to be able to tell at a glance when your client last had a perm, colour or trim
Hair condition	This will help you to identify any changes in the condition of the hair
Product used	This includes perming product, colours, shampoo and conditioners
Size of curler/rod, if perming	This will be useful next time you perm
Development time	Again, this will be useful next time, but you cannot rely on it completely. You will still need to check carefully each time you perm
Necessary precautions	Make a note of any precautions that you had to take
Finished result	The amount of curl, wave or lift. Did it turn out as you had expected? Was the client satisfied?
Recommended aftercare	Products that you recommended, or advice given to the client on maintaining her new hairstyle

Don't forget that any information which you keep on record is subject to the Data Protection Act 1998. You must treat all information confidentially and you must only use it for the purpose for which it was collected. This means that you can (and should) refer to it when planning your client's treatments, but if a shampoo representative asked for a list of your clients so that he could telephone them all to offer them cut-price shampoo, you could not give it to him.

Permanent waving faults and causes

The spider diagram below shows some perming faults that hopefully you will not experience during your hairdressing career.

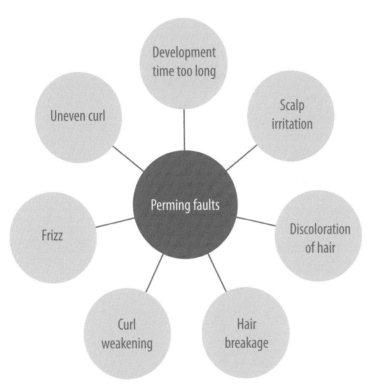

Problems with perming

Portfolio Activity

Once you have read through the causes below, you could discuss with your colleagues how to remedy each fault.

Development time excessively long

Owing to:
- wrong strength of lotion
- curlers too large
- sections too wide
- cold salon.

Scalp irritation
Owing to:
- cuts and abrasions on the scalp
- tension too tight (pull burns)
- too much lotion applied
- lotion too strong.

Discoloration of the hair

Owing to:

- incompatible chemicals used on the hair
- metal tools used
- incorrect selection of perm lotion.

Hair breakage

Owing to:

- too much tension
- twisted rubbers
- over-processing
- lotion too strong
- rubbers too tight.

Curl weakening

Owing to:

- incorrect neutralising process
- incorrect lotion selection
- incorrect development time
- rods too large.

Frizz

Owing to:

- lotion too strong
- rods too small
- over-processing.

Uneven curl across the whole head

Owing to:

- uneven sections taken
- root drag when winding
- not combing each section thoroughly when placing in the rod
- uneven tension
- uneven application of lotion
- incorrect use of end papers
- leaving some meshes of hair out of the rods by not tucking all hair around rod.

Perming Know How

1 Traditional alkaline perm lotions have a pH of approximately
a 10.0
b 12.0
c 9.5
d 7.5.

2 How many stages of the perming process are there?
a 5
b 2
c 4
d 3

3 If you are not sure whether a client's hair should be permed, you should:
a always refuse to perm
b take a test curl
c carry out the perm, but warn the client
d send the client to another salon.

4 Which bonds are broken during the perming process?
a sulphur bonds
b disulphide bonds
c hydrogen bonds
d oxygen bonds

5 PPE is a regulation to protect:
a you
b your client
c your salon
d the staff.

6 Which test should be carried out to determine the optimum rod size to be used?
a elasticity test
b development test curl
c incompatibility test
d pre-perm test curl

7 What is the main reason for a pre-perm treatment?
a to make the hair smell nice
b to detangle the hair
c to even out porosity
d to keep the hair moist during perming

8 During consultation, you notice that your client has a sore scalp. Do you:
  a continue with the perm
  b ask the client to seek medical approval
  c apply a barrier cream to the sore areas
  d suggest a scalp treatment and a perm when the scalp appears to be less sore?

9 In basic sectioning, how many sections do you divide the hair into?
  a 9
  b 7
  c 3
  d 5

10 What is the maximum amount of time that perm lotion should be left on the hair?
  a 25 minutes
  b 15 minutes
  c 20 minutes
  d 30 minutes

Kelly's Problem Page

Dear Kelly

A client came in the other day and asked for the telephone number of one of my other clients. They had apparently met at the salon a few weeks earlier, and she wanted to invite her to a coffee morning. My manager said that I could not give it to her. My client was a bit annoyed, and I felt awkward. What should I do if this happens again?

Kelly replies:

This is an embarrassing situation, isn't it? However, your boss was right and although your client may have been annoyed at the time, I am sure that she appreciated your position.

If it happened again, you could offer to telephone your client to ask if she minds you giving out her number or ask her to contact the client who wanted to invite her round. If she agreed, you could give out the number and everybody would be happy!

Dear Kelly

I have a client who always wants a tight curly perm but I think that it makes her look older. I have tried to suggest that she tries something different, but she says she likes her present style because she can wash it and forget it. I wish I could persuade her. Apart from anything else, I'm quite ashamed of people knowing that I turn her out looking like that!

Kelly replies:

Perhaps you could collect some magazines showing styles that would suit your client. If she likes a 'wash-and-go' style, she might have a busy lifestyle so don't try to persuade her to adopt a style that takes a lot of upkeep.

Don't tell her that a new style would make her look younger – that is as good as telling her that she looks older than her years now. Try pointing out the positive benefits of a new style.

If, despite all your efforts, she still wants to keep the style, remember that she is the client after all and it is her hair. As for being ashamed of turning out the client with a tight curly perm, don't be! As long as you are giving her a good perm that suits her hair type and lifestyle, you have nothing to be ashamed of. Whatever the style, healthy hair can look good!

Your Notes

Your Notes

Your Notes

UNIT5

COLOUR HAIR TO CREATE A VARIETY OF FASHION LOOKS

Introduction

This unit consists of one practical assignment, one written assignment and one written paper.

The practical assignment for this unit consists of two colouring tasks. You are required to colour two different clients' hair to create a variety of fashion looks. This practical assignment can be carried out on a man or woman, provided the clients chosen cover the range of colouring techniques and effects.

The written assignment will require you to have sufficient knowledge of how to colour a client's hair with varying requirements using a variety of techniques to achieve fashion looks and effects. You will be able to describe accurately the methods used and how choosing appropriate products and tools has helped you achieve this. You will need to understand the importance of taking into consideration factors that may influence the outcome of the colour.

The framework that you are working towards will determine whether the written paper is to be marked externally or internally.

To meet the criteria, you will use the skills that you have developed during your Level 2 work, specifically in unit numbers 206 (old standards) or H13 (new standards).

To complete the practical assignment correctly, you need to ensure that you are aware of the criteria against which you will be assessed. You must also make sure that you have the correct tools, products and equipment available within the salon to complete the tasks.

Colour hair to achieve different effects

Client 1 wants a colour fashion look that will lighten the whole head of hair. The client does not mind if you use colour or bleach.

Client 2 wants a look with a two-toned effect, with some parts lightened and some darkened.

When planning your assignments, you must select your clients carefully, and ensure that the look that you produce suits the client and her hair.

Hint: Client 2's requirements could be created using a variety of techniques, and it is entirely up to you how you create the desired two-tone effect. However, you are recommended to use high and low lighting.

You should be getting quite good at photography by now, because you should take some photos before, during and after your service, just as you did when you were cutting and perming.

The health and safety and other precautions that you need to take should be second nature by now.

Consider this

Before applying a colour to your client's hair, what precautions should you take to protect:

- your hands
- your client's skin
- your clothes
- your client's clothes?

The consultation procedure is very important before carrying out a colouring service. What information will you need to collect? Make a list and then compare it with the one below.

We think that you will need to consider the following factors.

- **Client's requirements** – These will determine the desired colour and the technique to be used to create the effect.
- **Hair texture** – This will help determine the absorption of colour. Fine hair will normally absorb colour more quickly than coarse hair.
- **Hair density** – This will affect the overall colour choice. For example, if your client has a mass of hair, you should try to persuade her against having a block colour. It will need to be broken up with the addition of another colour to eliminate any effect of solidness.
- **Hair condition** – You will need to carry out the necessary tests to ensure that the condition is suitable for colouring using the method you have chosen. If the hair is badly damaged, the result may be uneven.

- **Skin/scalp sensitivity** – Make sure that you carry out all necessary tests before you begin colouring.
- **Client's natural colour** – Check the client's base shade so that you predict the result of the colouring process.
- **Client's skin tone** – The target colour needs to blend with the skin tone. Your aim is to flatter the client's skin tone, and not to make her look washed out and pale.
- **Contra-indications** – Make sure the scalp is free of cuts, abrasions, infections and/or infestations.
- **Adverse conditions** – Can the colouring processes go ahead?

Hair colour theory

Yes, we're getting scientific again.

Tints are dyes that are used to add colour to the hair. This is the opposite of **bleaching** where the aim is to remove the hair colour.

Two major hair pigments are:
- black/brown **melanin** (sometimes called granular pigment)
- red/yellow **pheomelanin** (sometimes called diffuse pigment).

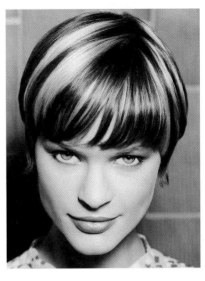

Hair colour can be used to create a variety of effects

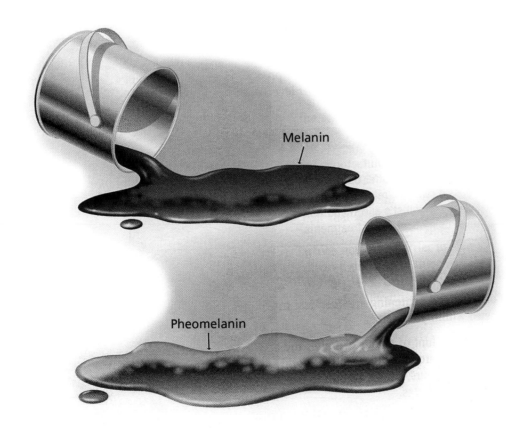

Melanin

Pheomelanin

Colour pigments

All natural colours are made up of a combination of colours. For example:

- **medium brown hair** has lots of brown and a little black, red and yellow
- **coppery red hair** has lots of red and yellow, but little brown and black
- **blonde** hair has lots of yellow and very little red and brown.

Hair pigments are found mostly in the cortex. The hair appears to be a certain colour to the eye because of the way in which the colour pigments absorb certain colours from the light falling on to it and reflect others. Only those colours that are reflected reach the eye, so a blue object appears blue because blue light is reflected and the other colours are absorbed. Black objects absorb light falling on them whilst white objects reflect all the light.

When tinting hair, you must also take the light quality into account. This can be a problem in that the mix of colours in artificial light is slightly different from that in daylight. The best way to achieve a true result is to look in natural daylight. If your salon has lots of large windows and white walls, then you should be able to see hair colour quite well. However, if the salon has poor lighting, then you may have to take the client over to a window and show them the true colours through a hand mirror.

Assessing your client's hair is a critical part of hair colouring, so try to organise your workstation so that you are not looking directly into the light. Glare can be both irritating and tiring on the eye.

Try assessing your own hair colour against different coloured backgrounds. The warmer the background, the warmer the colour of the hair will be. The darker the background, the more dull the appearance of your hair will be.

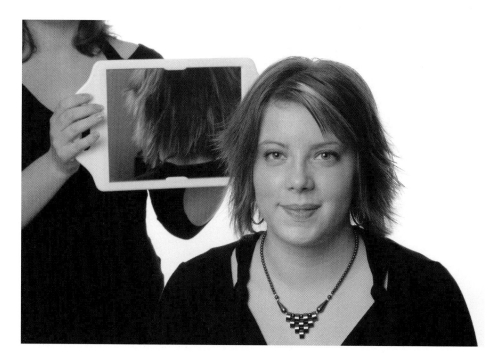

Mirror angles can be crucial in deciding hair colour

Natural hair colour

White hair – This contains no colour pigments at all. Remember, there is no such thing as grey hair; it is white hair mixed with naturally coloured hair.

For example:
- light brown hair and white hair looks salt and pepper
- dark brown hair and white hair looks steel grey.

Naturally coloured hair – This contains colour pigments found in the cortex. It is known as 'virgin hair', which means that it has never been artificially coloured.

When assessing the amount of white hair present in the base colour, you should part the hair down the centre of the head. If the first colour you see is white, the hair is more than 50 per cent white. If the first colour you see is base colour, the hair is less than 50 per cent white.

Use your colour chart to find an accurate match to your client's base shade. This analysis will determine the outcome of the colouring service.

Colour selection

We have discovered that human hair consists of two major groups of pigment (melanin and pheomelanin), which are deposited in the hair as it grows. Each head has a different distribution of these pigments and, depending on the reflection of light and the density of the hair, the base shades will be different on each head. If the hair is in good condition and has a smooth cuticle, it will reflect more light and appear lighter. If the hair is thick and abundant, it will be denser and appear darker. When analysing hair colour, you should take only a small section and this will enable you to assess the hair colour more successfully.

Skin tones

Younger clients generally have a fuller, plumper skin without lines and wrinkles. The skin of older clients has undergone changes in shape and texture and may also have lost colour. Very few older people have naturally rosy cheeks; any redness is often due to broken veins or cosmetic make up. Young people can therefore colour their hair most colours and look good (with the odd exception).

Dark or ashen colours can be very ageing to some older clients. They may wish to return their hair to its natural colour in order to look younger, but this is not usually successful. The colour they had then may not suit them now.

Hair in good condition

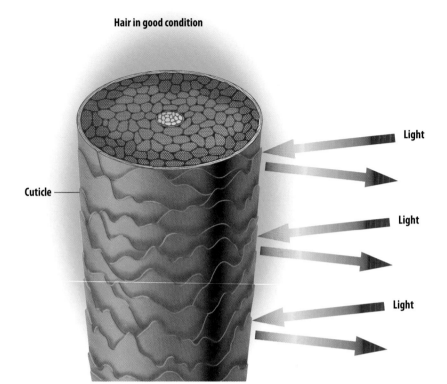

Cuticle

Light

Light

Light

Healthy cuticle scales reflect the light to show shiny, healthy hair. Cuticle scales in poor condition bounce the light back in all directions giving the hair a flat and dull appearance

Hair in bad condition

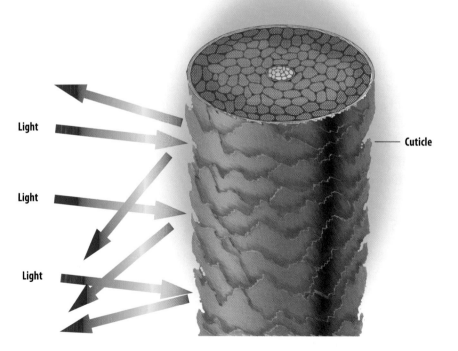

Cuticle

Light

Light

Light

Shade and depth of colour

You should have trained your eye to look at hair colours for two things:

- **The depth of colour** – This means how light or dark the hair is (very light blonde, light brown, etc.). This is called the base shade or level of colour.
- **The tone of colour** – This is the shade of colour on a particular depth (light ash blonde, light golden blonde, light warm brown, light copper blonde, etc.).

Remember, when using your shade chart, the label will show:
- the depth number
- the primary tone
- possibly, a secondary tone.

For example:

Depth	Primary tone	Secondary tone
5	4	6

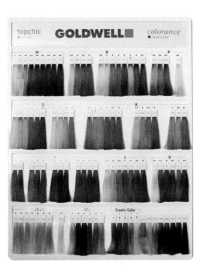

A shade chart

Portfolio Activity

This is a task for you to undertake with a colleague and you will need a colour chart.

First, one of you needs to select a hair shade from the chart. Then, without referring to the chart, describe the colour to your colleague. He or she must then select from the chart the colour that you are attempting to describe.

How long does it take you to describe a colour, and how accurate are you? Did your colleague select the right colour?

Hopefully this exercise has shown you how important a shade chart is. Your client may have a clear idea of what she wants, and you might have a clear idea of what you think would suit her, but you need to be sure that you both have the same thing in mind.

Follow these simple rules.
- Determine the level/base shade that you are starting with (use swatches from your colour chart to match the client's natural colour).
- Determine the level that you wish to achieve; you may want to lighten the hair or darken it, or you may wish to match the client's natural shade.
- Determine the required tonal value – does your client want warm, neutral or cool tones?
- Determine the strength of peroxide required, and the appropriate application method.

Types of colour

The colouring products that you use will be determined by the manufacturer's range that is used in your salon. This may include the following colouring products.

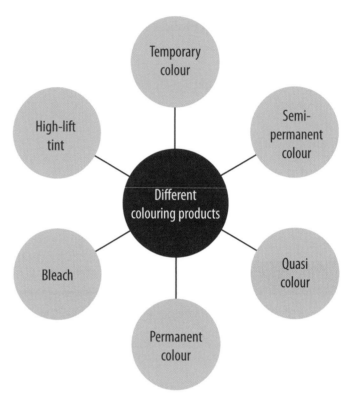

Hair may be coloured with a variety of products

Whichever range you use, you will probably find that it includes:

■ **Temporary colour**: including colour mousse/setting lotion, hair mascaras, etc. These colours will stain and coat the cuticle by adding large molecules, which will last only until the hair is next shampooed.

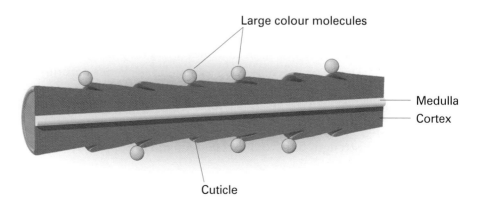

Temporary colour molecules coat the cuticle with a colour

- **Semi-permanent colour:** for example Colour Fresh, Hybrid, etc. These colours should last for between 4 and 8 washes, and should contain no peroxide. The colour molecules are small and large, allowing them to stay trapped within the cuticle for longer. These colours are not recommended for use on hair with a large percentage of white, because they are not intense enough to create depth.

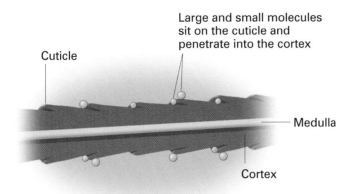

Semi-permanent colour molecules stain the cuticle

- **Quasi colour:** for example Colour Sync, Dia Colour, Colorance, etc. These colours contain small molecules that are trapped tight in the cuticle with a slight penetration into the cortex. They last between 15 and 20 washes.
- **Permanent colour:** peroxide is mixed with the colour to allow penetration into the cortex and to change the hair colour permanently. This colour will last until it grows out.

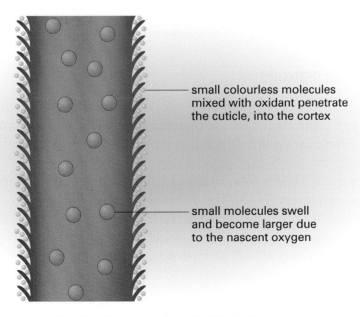

The effect of permanent colour on the hair structure

- **Bleach:** peroxide is mixed with the bleach, which will allow penetration into the cortex. This process has the opposite effect to permanent colouring. It removes the natural pigment (the process is called oxidisation). This will permanently lighten the colour of the hair, and the amount of lift will depend on the strength of peroxide and the development time.

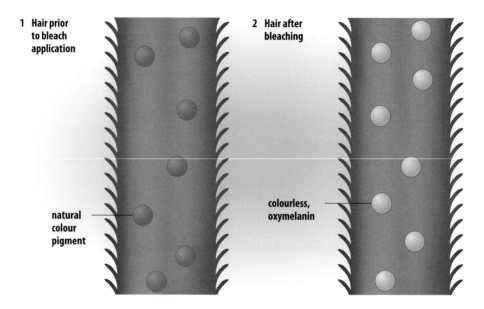

1 Hair prior to bleach application

2 Hair after bleaching

natural colour pigment

colourless, oxymelanin

The effect of bleaching on the hair structure

- **High-lift tint:** all manufacturers offer a high-lift range. This product is similar to bleach, but is much kinder to the hair. It will lift colour from the hair and lighten it, but it also enables the addition of tones. However, this product does not have the lifting power of bleach, and if you require more than five shades of lift, it will not be any use. This is a permanent product, and will last until it grows out or is cut out.

Hydrogen peroxide

Hydrogen peroxide is an agent that releases oxygen. The oxygen can then bind to the hair pigments and change the natural colour or, during neutralising a perm, rebuild the disulphide bonds in the hair to 'fix' the process.

Hydrogen peroxide is colourless and odourless and looks very much like its close relative water (H_2O). The difference is that hydrogen peroxide has an 'extra' atom of oxygen in its molecule, making it H_2O_2. Due to the 'extra' atom of oxygen, hydrogen peroxide is classed as an unstable substance as it decomposes spontaneously to form water and oxygen ($H_2O + O$). Stabilisers are added during manufacturing to avoid the loss of oxygen during storage. However, during colouring, bleaching and neutralising, the decomposition of the hydrogen peroxide is necessary as the newly formed oxygen – nascent oxygen – does all of the work.

It is essential that you consider the following factors that would rapidly break down the hydrogen peroxide.

- **Dust** – Tiny particles of dust in the air can cause rapid breakdown of hydrogen peroxide. To prevent this ensure that the top of the container is replaced immediately after use.
- **UV light and heat** – These accelerate the breakdown and, as both are present in sunlight, hydrogen peroxide should never be placed in direct sunlight. A dark, cool storage place is recommended.
- **Alkalis** – These are soluble substances that produce solutions with a pH above 7. Alkalis are deliberately used to speed the release of oxygen in hydrogen peroxide.

Peroxides come in the following strengths:

Peroxide strength	Use
10 volume/3%	Deposit colour only on natural or decolourised hair. Used for refreshing the mid-length and ends
20 volume/6%	Up to two levels of lift. Used for grey coverage and brighter fashion reds on natural hair
30 volume/9%	Up to three levels of lift
40 volume/12%	Up to four levels of lift. Use double developer with high-lift series for up to five shades of lift

Make sure that you follow manufacturer's instructions when preparing and mixing your colour. Some colorants are mixed in a 1:1 ratio, for example, 30 ml of oxidant to 30 ml of colour. However, others, such as high-lift tints, may be mixed on a 2:1 ratio, for example, 60 ml of oxidant to 30 ml of colour.

Occasionally within your salon you may discover that you have run out of the required peroxide strength and have no more in stock. In this instance you would need to dilute the peroxide strength that you have to the correct strength.

When diluting peroxide it is best to use distilled water along with liquid (not cream) peroxide. This will provide you with the correct consistency. For example, if you have 40 vol (12%) but need 20 vol (6%):

$\frac{20}{40} = \frac{2}{4} = \frac{1}{2}$ therefore you would need 1 part of peroxide to 1 part water.

If you had 40 vol (12%) but needed 30 vol (9%):

$\frac{30}{40} = \frac{3}{4}$ therefore you would need 3 parts of peroxide to 1 part water.

Quick tip

Always ensure that you are aware of the mixing procedure required prior to carrying out your colour.

Methods of colouring

You can achieve a variety of effects using different methods of application. Here are some ideas of what you can do.

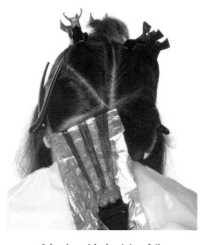

Colouring with aluminium foil

Aluminium foil – This is used mainly for weaving or slicing. The foil is used to wrap the hair in a similar way to Easi Meche packets. If they are applied correctly, the foils provide a much firmer method, as they eliminate the slipping that can occur with packets. They also allow you to get closer to the root. More than one colour can be used with this method.

Colour wraps – These are adhesive strips to which the hair will stick, allowing neat control. They are used for block colour and slicing. More than one colour can be used with this method.

Easi Meche – These are packets which open and have an adhesive blue line at the top on which the hair is placed. Once the colour is applied, the packet is closed. There is a tendency for the packets to slip, and seepage can occur. The blue line is the guide up to which the colour may be applied. More than one colour may be used.

Highlighting caps – These cannot be used for Level 3 assessments. A cap is used to create multi-lightening, and is best used when working with one colour only.

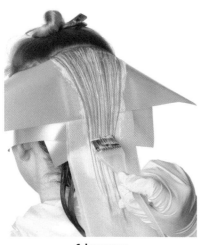

Colour wraps

Dappling – This is also called shoe shine or frosting. This method involves applying colour or bleach to the tips of the hair. It is mainly used on short hair, and can be done freehand or by using a piece of foil onto which the colour is placed. You then lightly rub or shine over the tips.

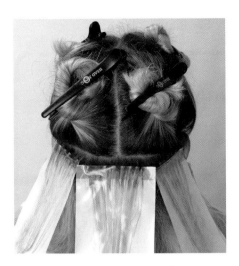

Easi Meche can be used to apply colour

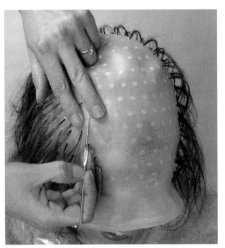

A highlighting cap

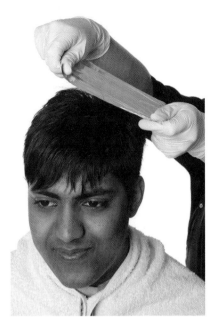

Dappling

Quick tips for fashion colouring techniques

- Introduce clients to colour gradually. Once they have gained confidence they will be more aware of the effects that can be created and will become more adventurous.
- Use colour as an extension of your client's personality.
- Ensure that you are comfortable with the colour manufacturer that your salon uses before experimenting too much.
- When using foils, Easi Meche or colour wraps, you should constantly monitor the process by checking for seepage at the roots. Colour will expand in this area due to the body heat escaping from the scalp.
- Ask for assistance when using two or more methods on one application as monitoring development time is essential – it may take one person over an hour to apply. You may need fresh tint throughout to ensure an even colour result.
- When mixing your colours, ask for assistance to ensure minimum wastage.
- Always advise your client on the correct aftercare to keep the colour looking at its best.

Portfolio Activity

For each of the following clients, state:

- any pre-care given or advised (include testing, hair condition, etc.)

- the chosen colour and why it was chosen

- peroxide strength

- sequence of application, e.g. roots then ends, or ends then roots

- development time for each stage.

Client 1 has shoulder-length, layered hair with a natural base shade of 6. She has applied semi-permanent colours to her hair in the past. She requires a shade lighter than her natural shade, and would like some warmth added but does not want her hair too red.

Client 2 has short hair with a base shade of 9.3. Her hair is about 30% grey and has a re-growth of about 2.5 centimetres (1 inch). She requires a darker colour as her hair has lifted in the sun and she would like a shade of 6. She also wishes to remove the warm tones from her hair.

Client 3 has a one-length bob with a natural base shade of 4. She has no previous colour on her hair which is 70% grey.

Client 4 has a mid-length, choppy style with a natural base shade of 3. She has previously had semi-permanent colours on her hair. She requires a vibrant violet glow to her hair and does not mind how bright the effect is.

Client 5 has short hair with a natural base shade of 9. Her hair has been coloured medium copper blonde and has about 5 centimetres (2 inches) of re-growth.

Client 6 has long, layered hair with a base shade of 10.1 (a very flat colour). Her hair is over 50% grey. She requires the grey to be covered and warmth added but does not wish her hair to be much darker.

Client 7 has thick, mid-length hair with a base shade of 8.3. Her hair is 40% grey. She requires a lighter effect although not necessarily full head. She would like the lightest blonde possible, but the condition of her hair will eliminate the use of bleach.

Client 8 has a long, one-length style with a base shade of 6. She requires lights for a sun-kissed look but does not wish her hair to go lighter than a base of 9. She also does not want her hair to look too gold but would be happy with beige.

Colour faults and causes

The spider diagram on page 153 shows some problems that can occur with colouring.

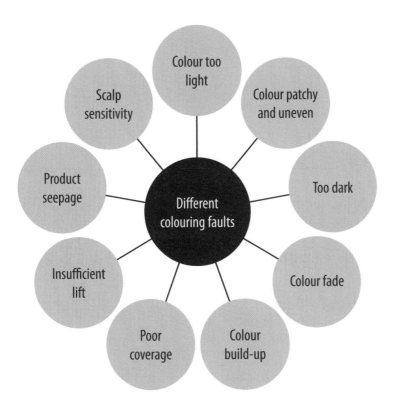

Problems with colouring hair

Colour too light
Owing to:

- wrong colour selection
- peroxide strength being too high
- under-processing.

Patchy and uneven colour result
Owing to:

- uneven application
- under-processing
- incorrect mixing of colour
- overlapping of application on original colour, causing build-up
- uneven porosity along the hair shaft.

Colour too dark
Owing to:

- wrong colour selection
- porous hair condition which will accept colour quicker
- over-processing.

Colour fade

Owing to:

- under-processing
- wrong colour selection
- wrong strength of peroxide
- porous hair.

Colour build-up

Owing to:

- overlapping during application
- combing through with tint unnecessarily.

Poor coverage on resistant hair

Owing to:

- wrong colour selection
- incorrect sequence of application
- wrong selection of peroxide
- not enough product used
- insufficient development time.

Insufficient lift

Owing to:

- wrong strength of peroxide
- natural base shade being too dark for the chosen colour
- insufficient development time
- wrong quantities of peroxide and colour mixed.

Product seepage

Owing to:

- too much product being applied
- colour being applied too close to the edge of the packet
- insufficient monitoring of development
- product being too runny.

Scalp sensitivity

Owing to:

- skin test not being carried out
- allergy to colour product
- peroxide strength being too high
- over-use of chemicals on the scalp.

Portfolio Activity

Listed on pages 153–4 are some colouring faults that we hope that you will not face during your hairdressing career. Now you have read through the causes, you can discuss with your colleagues how to remedy each fault.

Key Skills Activity Communication 2.1a

If you have this discussion with your colleagues, it could give you evidence for Key Skills Communications C2.1a. Don't forget to ask your group to write a witness statement, showing your contribution to the discussion, and don't forget to write a witness statement for them, which they can use for their evidence. Ask a tutor or assessor to watch the discussion, and ask for his or her assessment on how you met the criteria.

Colouring Know How

1 List two methods of colouring that allow penetration into the cortex.

2 Why is the porosity of the hair an important factor when colouring?

3 List the four rules for colour selection.

4 What are the three primary colours?

5 What makes a colour process quicker at the root area?

6 Which colour combination produces brown?

7 What are the two natural hair colours?

8 How do you assess the percentage of grey present in the hair?

9 What is the purpose of your colour chart?

10 With the aid of simple diagrams, describe the effects of the colour molecules on the hair shaft when using temporary, quasi and permanent colours.

Kelly's Problem Page

Dear Kelly

A new client came into the salon last week, and asked for a colour. I explained that I would have to do a sensitivity test first, but she said that she was in a terrible hurry, and that she did not have time to wait for the test.

I knew that my manager would be furious if I gave a colour without testing first, so I refused to do the colour. The client said that if she could not have the colour, she would not bother to have any treatment at all. Later that day, she came back, having had her hair coloured and cut in a different salon. She said that they had not insisted on a sensitivity test, and that she would be going to them in future.

I feel that I have lost a good potential client. What should I have done?

Kelly replies:

You did exactly the right thing. Nine times out of ten, a sensitivity test is negative, but on the tenth occasion, the test could well avert a disaster.

All reputable salons will have a rule that new clients must have sensitivity tests before colouring, perming or other chemical treatments are carried out. This might upset some clients, who are keen to have their hair done now and do not want to wait, but those same clients would not be too happy if you did not do the test, and something went wrong.

You probably won't see the client again – until the new salon cuts one corner too many. Then she might come back to ask you to repair the damage. If that happens, I'm sure you will be very helpful, and won't say 'I told you so' however much you might want to.

Kelly's Problem Page

Dear Kelly

A client has told me that she wants to change her hair colour. She said that she used to have a fabulous colour at the salon she went to before she moved to this area. She couldn't remember the name of the colour, but she knew what range it came from, and it isn't a range we stock. I showed her our colour chart, but she said the colour she wanted wasn't there. I explained that we could mix more than one colour to get what she wanted but I would need to know the exact colour she had in mind.

She's coming back this week to have the colour, and I don't want her to be disappointed. Have you any ideas that could help?

Kelly replies:

A couple of things spring to mind. First of all, you could try to obtain a colour chart from the range she mentioned. Then she could point out the one she wants. Alternatively, why don't you ring her previous stylist? Professional hairdressers know that clients move to other salons occasionally, and in your client's case, she moved because she left the area. The hairdresser could tell you if one colour, or a mixture, was used.

Whatever you do, don't guess! It's so difficult to describe a colour exactly, and it may be that your client remembers the colour differently to the way it really looked.

If you can't find the colour your client remembers, carry out a consultation as you would with any client wanting a new colour, and narrow down the possibilities until you come up with the perfect solution. I'm sure she'll love it.

Your Notes

UNIT6

STYLE HAIR TO CREATE A VARIETY OF FASHION LOOKS

Introduction

This unit consists of one practical assignment, one written assignment and one written paper.

The practical assignment for this unit consists of four tasks. You are required to carry out a range of styling and dressing techniques. This practical assignment can be carried out on a man or woman, provided the clients chosen cover the range of styling and drying techniques and effects.

The written assignment requires you to have sufficient knowledge of how to style a client's hair with varying requirements, using a variety of techniques to achieve fashion looks and effects. You will need to be able to describe accurately the methods used and how choosing appropriate products and tools and equipment has helped you achieve this. You will need to understand the importance of taking into consideration factors that may influence the outcome. The framework that you are working towards will determine whether the written paper is to be marked externally or internally.

To meet the criteria, you will use the skills that you have developed during your Level 2 work, specifically in unit numbers 203 (old standards) or H10 (new standards).

To complete the practical assignment correctly, you need to ensure that you are aware of the criteria against which you will be assessed. You must also make sure that you have the correct tools, products and equipment available within the salon to complete the tasks.

Preparation

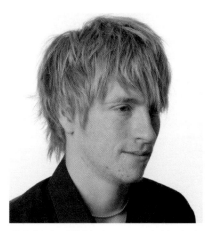

Hair dried and finished to create a fashion look

Client 1 wants you to dry and finish his hair to create a fashion look. The client would like the hair to be blow dried or finger dried.

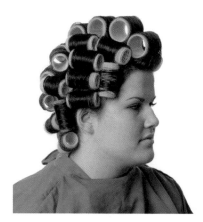

Hair being set

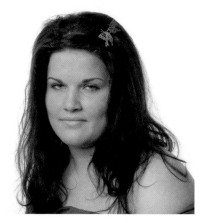

Hair dressed and dried to create a fashion look

Client 2 wants her hair to be set, dried and dressed into a fashion look. She is happy for you to use any type of roller or any other setting tool, but would like a wet set, as dry sets do not last in her hair.

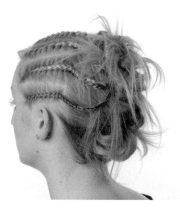

Long hair dressed into a fashion look

Client 3 wants her long hair dressed into a look that includes plaiting, braiding or knots.

Quick tip

Don't forget the photographs, and don't forget the health and safety precautions that you must take.

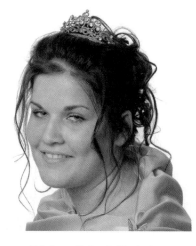

Hair dressed into a fashion look

Client 4 wants her hair dressed in a look that incorporates rolls, twists or curls.

You will need to carry out the usual consultation process with each client, and you will need to collect the information outlined below.

- **Client's requirements** – Is the style achievable? Will it suit your client?
- **Hair texture** – This will affect the choice of style. Is the texture suitable for the chosen style? Fine hair will need increased body and movement, and coarse hair requires firmer control. How much natural movement has the client's hair got? Is it curly or straight?
- **Hair length** – Is the hair long enough to achieve the style? On the other hand, is it too long? Longer hair will probably need larger rollers, depending on the amount of movement required. Shorter hair needs smaller rollers to achieve movement. Is the hair layered or one length?
- **Hair density** – The amount of hair will influence your choice of blow styling or setting technique.
- **Growth patterns and curl patterns** – The natural movement will help determine the best direction in which to blow dry or set the hair. If the hair is naturally wavy, you will need to add less curl than if the hair is straight.
- **Contraindications** – Is the scalp free of cuts, abrasions, infections and infestations?
- **Adverse conditions that may affect the outcome** – For example, alopecia.

Quick tip

In Unit 1, we looked at the way in which you should carry out a consultation. This might be a good time to refresh your memory.

Portfolio Activity

This activity should be placed in your portfolio under Unit 6, and it also provides key skills evidence.

Your best friend lives in Jersey, and is coming to England to get married in three months' time. She has asked you to do her hair, and that of the bridesmaids, for the big day. She is having no adult bridesmaids, just the four-year-old twin nieces of the bridegroom.

Your friend has very fine, wavy, shoulder-length hair, and she will be wearing a veil that fixes to the back of her head. She has written to you to ask you to suggest suitable styles for her type of hair. She would like to wear her hair up.

Her two young bridesmaids have thick, chin-length hair which they usually wear in a straight bob. She also wants you to make some suggestions about suitable ways of 'dressing up' their hair.

1 What other information would you need before you could recommend a suitable style? Think of the questions you would need to ask – you can choose your own answers.

2 Look through hairdressing magazines and other sources and find four styles that you think would suit your friend, and two that would suit her bridesmaids. Cut out pictures of each style and add a caption to each describing the style, and listing the reasons why you are recommending it.

3 Write a letter to your friend explaining why it is important that she has a trial run of the hairstyle before the wedding day.

4 Your friend is going to the Seychelles for her honeymoon – lucky girl! In her letter to you, she mentions that she hasn't got a clue what the weather there will be like in June. Using at least *two* sources of evidence, obtain information on the climate of the Seychelles, find out where the islands are located, summarise important local customs, currency used, and any other information you think your friend might like to have. Write a note to slip in with the letter, summarising your findings. You could also add some pictures.

When styling hair, either by blow drying or setting, you must first ensure that you have all the necessary tools available.

When blow drying, the length of hair will dictate the size of the brush that you choose. In the same way, the length of hair will dictate the size of roller when you are setting hair.

Always ensure that you have a clean and tidy workstation before your service starts. Place all your tools on your section or trolley. This will not only look professional, but helps to make sure that the service proceeds smoothly and no time is wasted.

You should have an extensive knowledge of the products available for use in your salon. You must consider the effects of different products on different types of hair. When styling and dressing, you should be looking for products that will help you to achieve the desired outcome. You want to ensure the maximum hold for your client, and this will obviously be influenced by whether your client wants a special occasion style or an everyday look.

Remember that if your client wants a special occasion hairstyle, it is always advisable to carry out a trial run first. This prevents problems arising on the day of the occasion, when time may be at a premium. Don't forget that you need to take into account the type of dress that your client will be wearing. You must also make sure that your client is aware of the cost of her special hairstyle. Negotiating this at the very start will prevent embarrassment on the day.

Dry and finish hair to create fashion looks

Blow drying

This involves drying damp hair into the required position with the aid of combs, brushes and a hand-held dryer. You can create a range of different effects by blow drying.

Quick tip

You need to make sure that the products are suitable for the client's scalp. If there are any adverse conditions, you do not want to irritate them.

Quick tip

Remind your client to wear a dress or top that does not have to be taken off over her head when she comes to the salon for her special style. It sounds obvious, but not everybody thinks of it.

You can create waves by using small radial heat retaining brushes:

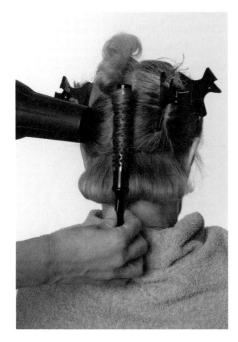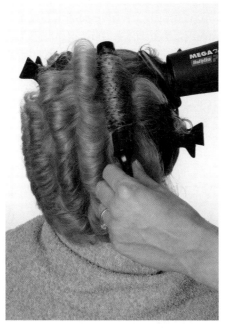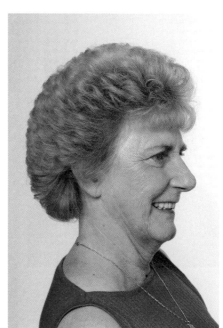

Creating waves by blow drying with a small brush

You can create a smooth, sleek effect with the use of a large radial heat-retaining brush, or Denman, or a paddle brush. You could use heated brushes or tongs once your blow dry is complete to achieve the final shape.

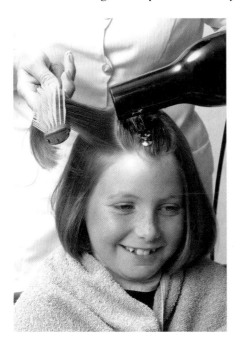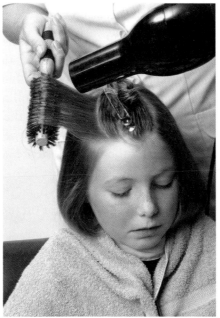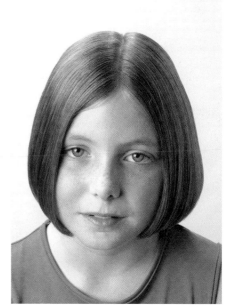

Creating a smooth, sleek effect

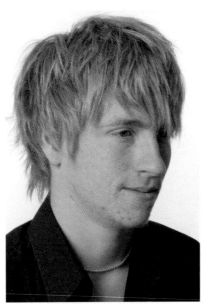

Finger drying will encourage natural movement in the hair

You can finger dry the hair to encourage any natural movement in the hair. You use your hands to manipulate the hair into the required direction.

This may simply involve scrunch/natural drying, but you may need the addition of a diffuser. This attaches to the end of the hand-held dryer and helps to diffuse the airflow from a strong to a gentle one, to produce an even flow.

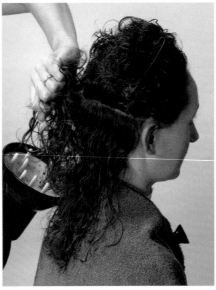

Scrunch drying hair with a diffuser

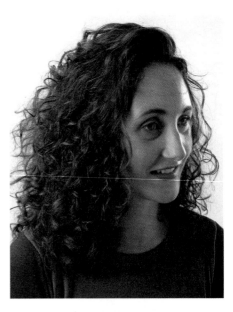

The finished result

Blow drying techniques

- Your dryer should be positioned down the hair shaft, from roots to points, to help keep the cuticle scales flat.
- Keep the dryer moving to avoid burning the client's hair or scalp.
- Don't overstretch the hair by pulling too hard.
- Lift the hair up when removing the brush, to prevent tangling.
- Don't have the heat on the dryer set too high.
- Don't overdry the hair. If you are not happy with the shape, wet the section and start again.

Remember: incorrect use of heat on the hair can cause:

- unnecessary damage to the hair
- burns to the scalp
- hair breakage
- discoloration of the hair.

The blow dry that you would be expected to produce at Level 3 would be at a more advanced level than the basic style that you produced when undertaking your Level 2 qualification.

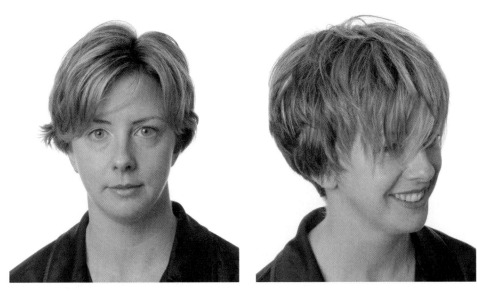

Blow drying to create a fashion look

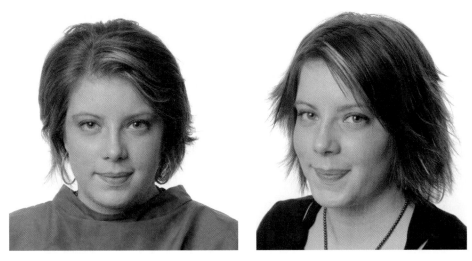

Drying a short cut

Set and dress hair to create fashion looks

Setting and pin curling

When setting both wet and dry hair, there are three things that you must remember:

1   **Sectioning** – Make sure that your section is of the correct width and depth. If it is too big, the roller will be placed incorrectly and the result will be unsatisfactory. The section should be slightly narrower than the roller, and slightly smaller in depth than the roller.

2   **Tension** – Ensure even tension and even distribution to make sure that you produce a uniform result.

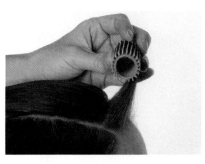

Take a section that is slightly narrower than the
length of the roller and no deeper than the
width of the roller

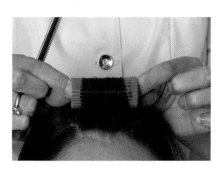

Good even tension is essential

3   **Angle** – The angle at which you hold the hair when winding will
     determine the amount of root lift that you will achieve. Good root lift
     should be produced by holding the hair at a 90-degree angle from the
     head. This will ensure that the roller will sit upon its own root area. For
     some fashion styles, you may want to create root drag to produce little
     or no root lift.

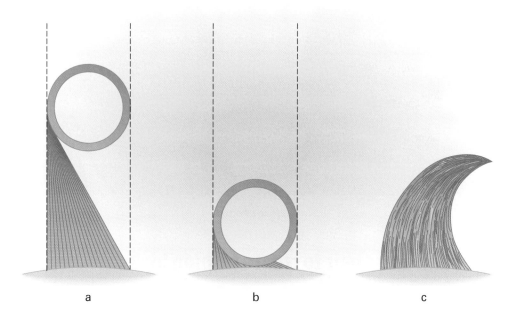

a   b   c

Hair wound to sit on its own base

Setting techniques

There are three different types of wind:

1   **Channel** – This is a uniform layout, beginning at the front hairline.
     Direct the rollers in a channel row down the centre of the head. Work
     the crown area downwards, at either side of your centre section. Finish
     by placing another set of rollers at the side of the head.

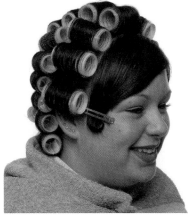

Channel technique

2   **Brickwork** – The rollers are placed in a brickwork formation, the same as a brick wall layout. Put one roller at the front section, take the next section from the middle of the first roller, and continue working down the head until the set is complete.

3   **Directional** – The rollers should be placed in the direction that you want the hair to be dressed.

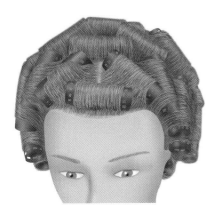

Brickwork technique

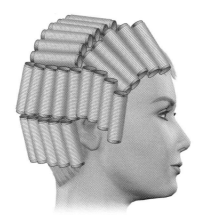

Directional winding

These winds can be used in combination, using more than one technique to achieve the style you want.

Pin curling techniques

Pin curling is useful for shorter hair, for which roller setting might not be appropriate.

1   **Flat barrel curl** – This will lie flat to the head with an open centre. It will help to produce a curl which is from root to point. A clip will hold the curl in place. If flat barrel curls were placed with one row in one direction, and one row in the opposite direction and so on, a wave would be produced. Two rows in one direction and two rows in the opposite direction create a larger waved effect.

2   **Stand-up barrel curl** – This is formed on a similar basis as rollering, but without the roller. A clip will retain the lifted base and curl position.

3   **Clockspring curl** – This will also sit flat on the head with a closed centre. It produces a tighter curl effect on the points.

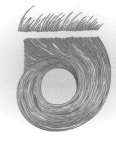

Flat barrel curl

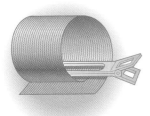

Stand-up barrel curl

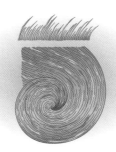

Clockspring curl

Finger waving

Finger waving is a method of setting which moulds the hair into an 'S' shape using the hands, a comb and clips to hold the shape. In horizontal, the waves will go from side to side. While this is a very old technique, it regularly appears in style books and on the heads of celebrities.

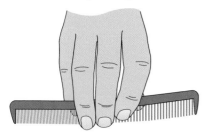

Finger waving

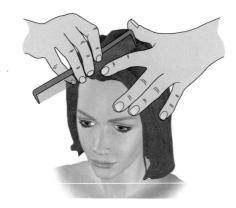

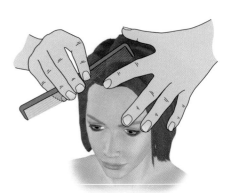

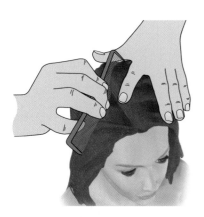

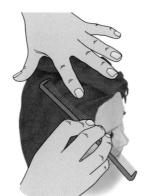

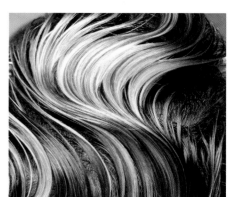

The finished result

> **Quick tip**
>
> Although it is not essential that you use all the above styling, blow drying or setting techniques, it is essential that you ensure that you have sufficient knowledge of the techniques that you could use to create different effects.

The point at which the hair changes direction is known as the crest. The height of the crest and the depth will depend on the amount of moulding with the fingers. Finger waving can be produced on straight or naturally wavy hair. However, it is less successful on naturally tight curls or permed hair.

Dress long hair

After all the planning and preparation, dressing is the process of adding the finishing touches to create the desired look. You may have produced movement, lift and curl through setting or blow drying, but without the correct finish, your style and skill will be wasted. It is this look that the client will take away from the salon.

You may need to brush the hair thoroughly to blend in waves, remove roller partings and eliminate the stiffness caused by products.

You may need to add some back brushing to create more lift and volume. By brushing backwards from the points to the roots, you will help bind the hair together to create a fuller shape. This technique is especially useful for fine hair.

If you want a firmer, stronger method of providing support and volume, you may need to add backcombing. This is applied deep to the scalp and produces a stronger effect. It is especially useful when you are putting long hair up.

Line and balance

Balance refers to the shape of the dressing in relation to the client's face, neck and head. The lines of the style should complement the wearer. Judging when the finished style is balanced requires practice and with the use of the mirror you can achieve a clearer all-round view to assess this. Dressing the hair close up limits the vision of the stylist to one area, so it is important to check the outline and shape in the mirror frequently to gain a clearer idea of where the style may need altering.

When styling is complete, stand away from the head and check the line and balance of the style at the front, sides and back of the head. First, look at the silhouette of the style, checking for obvious defects, then check the smoothness is correct. Next, check the edges of the hairline are neat and even to ensure they blend and complement the face and neck shape.

> **Quick tip**
>
> You should advise your client on how to remove backcombing/back brushing correctly. Incorrect removal can be very painful and damaging to the hair.

> **Quick tip**
>
> The final image will become what the stylist and the salon's reputation will be judged on; it is worth taking an extra few seconds to check that nothing mars the hairstyle.

> **Quick tip**
>
> Different mirror angles can help you to be sure that everything is right

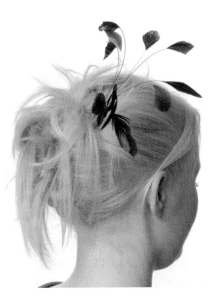

Hair has been styled using a combination of knots and twists. Added hair and feathers have been placed into the hair to add definition, colour and individuality

Hair has been styled using a combination of rolls and twists. Feather ornamentation has been carefully placed to add some contrast to the client's natural hair colour

Portfolio Activity

It is essential that your client is happy with the finished result. You are probably used to holding up the mirror behind your client and hearing her say, 'That's lovely, thank you'. Have you thought what you would do if the client said, 'No, sorry, I don't like it.'

What would you say in the following circumstances?

1 You have cut the client's hair, and she feels that it is too short.

2 You have put up the client's long hair, and she doesn't like the back view.

3 You have highlighted your client's hair and she is disappointed that there are fewer highlights than she would have liked.

Discuss this with your group and try to come to an agreement as to what you would do in each case. Then discuss what you could have done to have prevented it happening in the first place.

Write down what you have agreed and ask everybody else in the group to sign to confirm their agreement.

Physical changes during blow drying and setting

There are two types of bonds/cross linkages that are found in the polypeptide chains within the cortex:

1 Bonds that can be broken by water. Temporary bonds – hydrogen bonds and salt linkages.

2 A stronger type of bond that cannot be broken by water. Permanent bonds – disulphide bonds.

The first stage of blow drying or setting involves breaking some of the temporary bonds to reveal the hair in its natural unstretched state. This is known as alpha keratin.

The second stage involves drying and stretching the hair into its new temporary position. This is known as beta keratin. This process can be achieved through either blow drying or setting. You can make straight hair curly or curly hair straight. However, this will last only until the temporary bonds are broken again by the addition of water.

The effects of humidity

Our hair is hygroscopic, which means that it is able to absorb and retain moisture. The amount of moisture in the hair will affect the created style's durability. As the hair picks up moisture, the bonds will break down, allowing the hair to form into its natural alpha shape. The humidity, which is the moisture content of the air, will largely influence how long the style will be retained for. Careful selection of styling product will help eliminate the effects of humidity. Some products contain resin or plastics which coat the hair with a fine film to help prevent moisture from being absorbed into the hair.

Naturally straight hair becomes curly, changing alpha to beta keratin

Naturally curly hair becomes straight, changing alpha to beta keratin

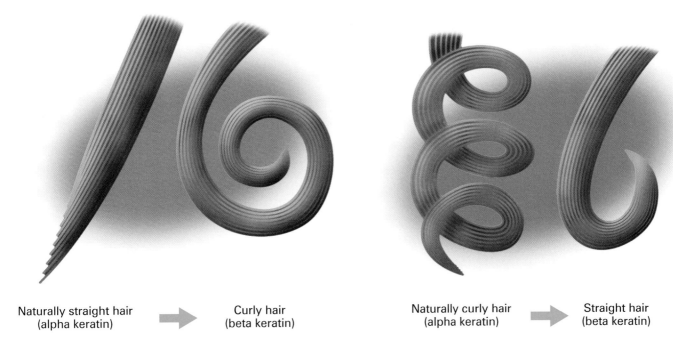

Naturally straight hair (alpha keratin) → Curly hair (beta keratin)

Naturally curly hair (alpha keratin) → Straight hair (beta keratin)

Straight and curly hair in natural and stretched states

Key Skills Activity Application of Number N2

In this unit, you have to style hair to create a variety of fashion looks. Some salons specialise in trendy hairstyles, some specialise in hairstyles for the older lady, and some work with a variety of clients and provide a variety of styles.

What sort of salon do you work in? You probably think you know, but let's try to get some evidence to back up your hunch.

1 You need information about your salon's clients over the past month, and the services with which they were provided. A good place to find this information could be the appointments book, but you can use another source if you can think of a better one.

2 Prepare a chart, listing services provided under various headings. The following headings are suggestions; you can add some or leave some out depending on your clientele:

cut and blow dry

cut and set

shampoo and set

perm

colour

highlights

long hair up.

3 Complete your chart, showing how many of each service you provided for each day of the month.

4 Work out the total number of services provided and calculate each service as a percentage of the total. For example, if you provided 100 services, split them up as follows:

> 30 cut and blow dries
>
> 15 cut and sets
>
> 5 shampoo and sets
>
> 3 perms
>
> 12 colours
>
> 25 highlights
>
> 10 long hair up.

The percentages would be:

> 30% cut and blow dries
>
> 15% cut and sets
>
> and so on.

Check your working to make sure that your calculations are correct.

5 Present your findings as:

> a pie chart
>
> a bar chart
>
> a scatter graph.

6 Write down how your findings will affect your opportunities to collect evidence for this unit.

This activity covers all the Application of Number key skills: N2.1.1, 2.1.2, 2.1.3, 2.2.1, 2.2.2, 2.3.1, 2.3.2, 2.3.3 and 2.3.4.

Check Your Styling/Dressing Hair Know How

1 What would be the result if too large a section was taken when placing a roller during setting?

2 What would be the result if you dressed the hair when it was not fully dry after styling?

3 What are the potential consequences of incorrect heat application on the hair?

4 What are the three different types of winding used in setting?

5 Why do you need to ensure even tension is applied during setting?

6 What type of hair is the pin curling technique useful for?

7 During finger waving, what is the name used for the point at which the hair changes direction?

8 What is the correct procedure for removing backcombing?

9 Which bonds are temporarily broken by water?

10 What effect does humidity have on the hair?

11 Why should the mirror be frequently used when dressing the hair?

Kelly's Problem Page

Dear Kelly

One of my regular clients is getting married next month and she wants me to put her hair up. She will be wearing a veil and a tiara, and she has asked me for some ideas on suitable styles.

I gave her a couple of bridal magazines, and she said that she would look through them and decide on a style that she likes. I said that I would book her in early on the wedding day, so that she wouldn't have to rush.

My boss interrupted, and said that we offer a 'wedding package' which brides should use. It is really expensive but the client agreed that she would use it. I will be getting married myself next year and know how expensive weddings are, so I was very embarrassed at my boss's 'hard sell'.

I thought of telephoning the client and telling her that she need not use the 'package' but I think my boss might be annoyed – all he thinks about is money. What should I do?

Kelly replies:

I know how you feel – weddings are expensive. However, are you sure that your wedding package is really a rip-off?

Most packages include lengthy consultations with the stylist, a 'trial run' before the big day to ensure that the chosen style suits the bride and that the veil and tiara are shown off to best advantage, as well as the exclusive services of a team of stylists for the bride and bridesmaids (and possibly the mother of the bride, too) on the wedding day.

The bride can be sure that she will leave the salon with her hair looking its best, in a style that complements her wedding outfit.

She could, of course, just book in on the morning to have her hair put up, but there would not be time to try out a number of different styles, and she would have to hope that the one she had chosen would work.

If the client seemed happy with the package to which she agreed, I suggest that you let things be, and concentrate on making sure that you give her the very best wedding hairstyle you can. Make sure that she gets her money's worth. Good luck!

Kelly's Problem Page

Dear Kelly

Last week, a client came in to have her hair put up, as she was going to a summer ball. She brought a photograph with her, but it was not suitable for her type of hair.

I tried to tell her that the finished effect would not be the same as the photo, and I suggested some changes that we could make so that the overall effect would be similar, but more suited to her hair.

She would not listen and insisted that I should copy the photo. With the help of a lot of gel, hairspray, tongs (and luck!), I managed to get it looking reasonably like the picture, but I was not happy because I knew that it would not last.

The following day, the client stormed back into the salon and demanded to see the manager. She said that her hair was starting to fall down even before she got to the ball. She said that it looked such a mess that she went into the ladies' toilet and tried to brush it out, but because I had used so much gel and hairspray it looked awful when she brushed it out. She said that she went home early and that I had spoiled her evening.

My boss listened to my side of the story and she managed to calm the client down somehow. I feel awful though because the client didn't have a good evening at the ball. What should I have done?

Kelly replies:

Well, you tried. If a client just won't listen and insists on an unsuitable style, it is very difficult to persuade her.

You did the right thing by suggesting suitable alternatives that would give the same overall effect. If you knew that you would have to use a lot of product on the hair, you could have pointed out to the client that if the style did not last, the hair would not brush out successfully, and would probably have to be washed before it looked good again.

Just one more point – make sure that you stress to the client that it is the style that is unsuitable, not her hair. In other words, 'that style would not flatter you' is better than 'you've got the wrong sort of hair for that style'. If you tell somebody she has the wrong sort of hair, she might take it as a challenge and insist that she hasn't. Then you will end up struggling, just as you did with your client!

Kelly's Problem Page

Dear Kelly

I am not very good at putting hair up. I have tried but I really find it difficult. I find this quite upsetting because I have always been quite good at my work so far. I'm good at colouring and I am always booked up for weeks ahead with clients wanting cuts. I don't want to sound big-headed but I've got quite a reputation as a good cutter.

Now I dread the day when a regular client asks for her hair to be put up. What on earth will she think when I have to say that I can't do it?

Help, please!

Kelly replies:

Not everybody can be good at everything. You said that you are good at colouring and you are obviously a brilliant cutter. That doesn't mean that you don't have to bother learning how to put hair up; you will need a lot of practice but once you get the knack you will be able to do it.

It may never be the thing that you are best at but you will certainly learn how to do it to an acceptable standard. A hairdresser needs to master all techniques, not just those which he or she finds easy.

However, don't be afraid of telling a client that putting hair up is not your best point. If there is somebody in your salon who is an absolute whizz at it, you could always suggest that your colleague takes over for that part of the service. This is nothing to be ashamed of; it just means that you will be ensuring that your client receives the best possible hair style.

Kelly's Problem Page

Dear Kelly

We have a very good trainee in our salon, who is becoming excellent at blow drying hair. She is very reluctant to learn setting techniques and, to be honest, I don't blame her. Hardly anybody comes into our salon for a 'shampoo and set' (thank goodness). She has to learn setting techniques in her day-release class at college, but she is not enjoying it. I've told her that she just has to grit her teeth and get on with it, but have you got any tips on how she can get through this boring part of her training?

Kelly replies:

I don't want to sound harsh, but maybe if you were a little less negative, she would be too. Those clients who do venture into your salon for a set are every bit as important as the clients who have the trendy hairstyles you obviously prefer. Anyway, roller and setting techniques are not only used for 'shampoo and sets'. They are important when creating fashion styles, and if you went behind the scenes at a fashion show, you would be surprised by how many 'trendy' models have their hair in rollers.

Setting techniques are not always easy to learn. They can be quite complicated, and you need to select the appropriate technique to achieve the style you want. You should be encouraging your trainee to learn as much about this type of hairdressing as she can and to become as good at it as she is at blow drying.

Hairdressers have to produce all types of hairstyles, not just those which they personally like. A fully trained and expert hairdresser can turn their hand to any type of hair styling, even those which they do not use every day in the salon.

This does not mean that you cannot specialise. You can, of course, but not until you have mastered every technique.

Your Notes

Your Notes

Your Notes

SECTION3

EMPLOYMENT RIGHTS AND RESPONSIBILITIES

Introduction

If you are taking an Advanced Apprenticeship, you will also need to complete this Employment Rights and Responsibilities section. This section will help you to understand the rights and responsibilities that you have as an employee, and those that your employer has towards you. Even if you are not taking a Modern Apprenticeship, you will still need to know your rights and responsibilities as an employee, so you should complete the activities in this section.

This unit contains the information that you need and directs you to other sources of information. It also shows how this information relates to your own employment.

When you have completed all the activities in this section you should get them signed off by your employer and tutor.

Statutory rights and responsibilities

These rights and responsibilities relate to employees only and not to people who offer a service on a self-employed basis.

Contracts of employment

A contract of employment is a legally binding document that sets out the terms and conditions that relate to the relationship between you and your employer. A verbal agreement is just as binding as a written one.

Within two months of starting work with an employer, you are entitled to a written statement. This applies to full-time and part-time employees. The contents of a written statement are shown below.

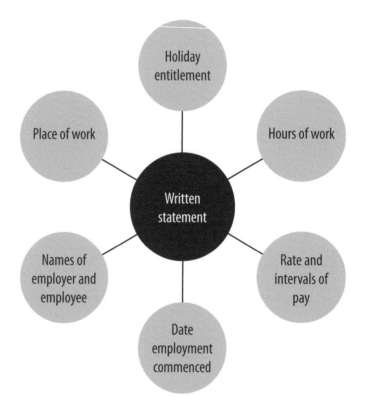

Contents of a written statement

Your company might refer you to other documents (such as a staff handbook) for information on sick pay, pension rights, disciplinary and grievance procedures and trade union rights. Any documents to which you are referred must be available to you in normal working hours.

Your employer might also add clauses referring to:

- the right to require you to undergo a medical examination, under certain circumstances
- the right to search
- confidentiality or fidelity.

Your contract of employment may be permanent or for a fixed term.

Altering your contract

Once your terms and conditions have been agreed, neither your employer nor you can vary them without consultation. There are a number of ways in which you and your employer might vary your contract.

Your contract can be altered:

- by agreement with you
- through negotiation and agreement with a recognised trade union, if the union has collective bargaining rights
- where a flexibility clause exists in the written statement that gives your employer the right to make reasonable changes
- by replacing the old contract with a new one which is agreed by both parties.

Terminating your contract

When you have completed one year's service, your contract of employment cannot be terminated unfairly. If your employer wishes to dismiss you they must give you a written statement of the reasons for the dismissal. Your company must follow its disciplinary/redundancy procedures, if these are in place. Even if the company does not have its own procedures, it must follow the ACAS guidelines, the main terms of which are as follows:

Written statement – Your employer must set out in writing the circumstances that have led them to consider dismissing you. They must send you a copy of the report and invite you to a meeting to discuss the matter.

Meeting – This must take place before any action is taken (unless you have been suspended). You must take all reasonable steps to attend the meeting. After the meeting, your employer must advise you of their decision and notify you of your right to appeal if you are not satisfied.

Appeal – If you wish to appeal, you must advise your employer and they must invite you to a further meeting. You must take all reasonable steps to attend this meeting. The appeal meeting does not have to be held before the disciplinary action or dismissal takes place. After the appeal, your employer must advise you of their decision.

Unfair dismissal

Some cases of dismissal are automatically considered unfair, and in these cases you do not need to complete one year's service before you are protected. Unfair reasons for dismissal include:

- sex, race or disability discrimination
- pregnancy, childbirth or taking maternity leave
- trade union membership, or refusal to belong to a union
- taking appropriate action for health and safety reasons
- acting as employee trustee of a pension scheme
- acting, or proposing to act, as an employee representative
- asserting a statutory right
- a refusal on the part of a protected shop worker to work on Sundays
- a refusal on the part of an employee to opt out of the Working Time Regulations 1998
- a 'qualifying disclosure' under the Public Interest Disclosure Act 1998 (also known as 'whistle blowing').

You have the right to take your case to an employment tribunal if you believe that you have been unfairly dismissed.

Key Skills Activity Communication C2.2

1 Find the following documents and put a copy into your portfolio.

a Your contract of employment.

b Your employer's grievance procedure.

c Any other documents to which your contract of employment refers.

Note: If your contract of employment refers you to a staff handbook, or similar file, do not take a copy for your portfolio. Instead, make a note of where it is kept and what arrangements are in place for you to read it.

2 Answer the following questions.

a What period of notice would you have to give if you wished to leave your employment?

b What is the name of the person to whom you would complain if you had a grievance?

c Are you paid weekly or monthly? On which day of the week, or date in the month, are you paid? Does your payment go straight into your bank account or are you paid by cheque?

d How many days' holiday per year are you entitled to?

e What arrangements does your employer have for paying you if you are away from work through illness?

Anti-discrimination

You have a legal right not to be discriminated against on the grounds of sex, race or disability, and this applies during the recruitment and selection process as well as whilst in employment.

Direct discrimination

Direct discrimination occurs when candidates or employees are excluded from consideration for employment, promotion or training on the grounds of sex, race or disability.

Indirect discrimination

Indirect discrimination can also occur, and this is less clear cut. If an employer sets conditions that can only reasonably be met by one sex or race and they cannot prove that there is an overriding business requirement for these conditions, that would be indirect discrimination.

Disabled employees

Employers have a duty to make reasonable adjustments to working practices and conditions in order that the needs of disabled employees can be met. Examples include changing the office layout to enable wheelchair access, or changing shift patterns to accommodate special requirements. However, if an employer can show that there are substantial reasons why a disabled person could not do a particular job, and there is no adjustment that could be made to accommodate the disabled person, then discrimination would not be unlawful.

Age

It is not currently illegal to discriminate on the grounds of age, although some jobs have lower age limits set by law.

Legislation

There are several Acts relating to anti-discrimination.
- The Equal Pay Act 1970
- The Sex Discrimination Act 1975
- The Race Relations Act 1976
- The Disability Discrimination Act 1995 (applies to all employers with 15 or more employees)

The following Acts and Regulations all refer to Employment Law.
- The Equal Pay Act 1970 (as amended)
- The Equal Pay (Amendment) Regulations 1983
- The Rehabilitation of Offenders Act 1974
- The Sex Discrimination Acts 1975 and 1986
- The Race Relations Act 1976
- The Employment Act 1989

- The Employment Relations Act 1999
- The Disability Discrimination Act 1995
- The Asylum and Immigration Act 1996
- The Police Act 1997
- The Data Protection Act 1998
- The Part-time Workers (Prevention of Less Favourable Treatment) Regulations 2002

Key Skills Activity Communication C2.2

Your company's equal opportunity policy will contain information relating to the company's employment practices. Find a copy of your company's equal opportunities policy and answer the following questions.

1 If you felt that you were being discriminated against in your workplace, what is the name of the person to whom you would report it?

2 If you were being discriminated against in your training centre or college, what is the name of the person to whom you would report it?

3 Disability is a wide-ranging term. Other than wheelchair users, can you think of two examples of disabilities? For each of these examples, what are the difficulties the person in question would have in working for your company and what arrangements could be made to improve things for him or her?

4 Give one example of an occupation that you believe would be exempt from the Sex Discrimination Act and say why.

Working hours and holiday entitlement

Working Time Regulations 1998 apply to all employers in the UK regardless of sector or size of organisation.

Working hours

Under these regulations you cannot be forced to work more than 48 hours per week unless you specifically agree to opt out.

The regulations also give an entitlement to rest breaks.

- Daily rest periods – workers are entitled to an 11-hour break in every 24-hour period in which they work.
- Weekly rest periods – workers are entitled to a break of 24 hours in every seven days. This can be averaged out over two weeks.
- Breaks during the working day – where a worker's day is longer than six hours, they are entitled to an uninterrupted break of 20 minutes during which they don't need to remain in the workplace.

Young people aged under 18 years are entitled to:

- a break of at least 30 minutes when they have worked for 4½ hours
- a free health assessment before starting night work and at appropriate intervals thereafter
- a daily rest of at least 12 hours
- a weekly rest break of at least 48 hours in a seven-day period.

Holiday entitlement

Under these regulations, all employees have a right to 20 days' holiday per year. This can include statutory holidays. An employee begins to accrue holiday rights as soon as their employment commences.

You must give your employer notice that you wish to take a holiday. This notice period should be at least twice as long as the holiday requested (e.g. two weeks' notice for one week's holiday).

Other leave

You have a legal right to time off work for public duties, such as jury service, but your employer does not have to pay you for this time.

Absence and sickness

Sickness

You have a right to Statutory Sick Pay (SSP) which will be paid by your employer in the same way and at the same time as your salary would have been paid. This is payable for periods of between four days and 28 weeks in any one period of incapacity.

Your employer may give you additional payments, and these should be specified within your contract of employment or in accompanying documentation.

Most employers allow their staff to provide a 'self-certificate' for the first few days of their illness, but a doctor's certificate will be required for longer spells of absence. Your employer must advise you of their requirements as part of your contract of employment.

Maternity leave

All women, regardless of length of service, are entitled to time off to attend antenatal care. The employer may ask for documentary proof (e.g. an appointment card or letter).

Women are entitled to 26 weeks' ordinary maternity leave, which cannot be started before the 11th week before the expected week of confinement (EWC). Women who have at least one year's service at the 11th week before the EWC are entitled to additional leave of up to 26 weeks, starting on the week of childbirth. It is illegal to allow a woman to return to work during the two weeks after the EWC. A woman must advise her employer at least 21 days before she begins maternity leave.

After additional maternity leave, the woman has the right to return to the same job, or one that is appropriate and no less favourable than her old job. After ordinary maternity leave, the woman is expected to return to her old job.

Key Skills Activity Communication C2.2

1 What are the arrangements for notification of sickness within your company?

2 How many days are you allowed to self-certify for before you need a certificate from your doctor?

3 How long do you have to be absent before SSP becomes payable?

4 Where could you find a self-certification form?

5 What is the minimum number of weeks of 'ordinary maternity leave' to which a woman is entitled following the birth of her child?

Data protection and access to personal information

Your company is entitled to keep records about your employment. The Data Protection Act 1998 gives you some protection against misuse of this data and covers both computerised and manual records.

Under this legislation, the information may be used only for the purpose for which it has been collected and may not be passed on to an unauthorised third party without your permission.

Data should be kept up to date and not retained for any longer than is necessary.

You have the right to read the data that your employer holds about you.

Key Skills Activity Communication C2.2

1 Where are your personnel records held, and who is responsible for ensuring that their contents are kept confidential?

2 Can you think of an example of an outside agency that would be able to ask your employer for information about you?

3 Why is it important that you advise your employer about changes in your personal circumstances (e.g. address, marital status, etc)?

4 To whom would you report such changes within your own organisation?

5 If you found something within your personnel record that was inaccurate, what steps would you take?

6 Do you have the right to see a colleague's personnel records?

Health and safety

During your induction, you should receive health and safety training from your employer. This section will make sure that you have understood the essential elements of health and safety.

Key Skills Activity Communication C2.2

1 Find the following documents, and put a copy into your portfolio.

a Your employer's health and safety policy.

b The health and safety policy of any college or training centre that you attend as part of your training.

2 After reading these documents, answer the following questions.

a Give two examples of health and safety regulations that apply to your workplace.

b Who is the 'nominated person' within your workplace who is responsible for health and safety arrangements? Give their name and job title, and say how they can be contacted.

c What arrangements are in place for evacuating the building in the case of fire? Who is responsible for checking that everybody is present?

d After the building has been evacuated, when may you return to the building?

Kelly's Problem Page

Dear Kelly

I have been working for my employer for over a year, but I have never been given a contract of employment. I asked my boss about this, but he said that he was a hairdresser, not a Personnel Manager, and he did not have time to worry about paperwork.

Does this mean that I do not have any employment rights?

Kelly replies:

No. You are entitled to a written statement of terms and conditions of employment, and your boss is breaking employment law by failing to provide you with one. The fact that he has not done so, however, does not mean that you have lost your rights.

Perhaps you could suggest to him that he asks his solicitor or accountant to draw up contracts for the staff. If all else fails, you could get further advice from the Citizens Advice Bureau, but it is always best to sort these things out informally, if possible.

Your Notes

Your Notes

SECTION 4: KEY SKILLS MAPPING GRID

The grids below set out the key skills criteria covered by the activities in this book. Some points to remember about key skills:

- You do not have to do every key skills activity, provided you do enough to cover the requirements of the examining board. If you have produced key skills evidence from other sources, simply select those activities that you need to fill the gaps in your evidence. Your tutor or assessor will be able to advise you about this.

- The activities can provide evidence to meet the criteria, but you must read the criteria, and ensure that the work you produce has sufficient depth and breadth.

Application of Number

Activity	N2.1.1	N2.1.2	N2.1.3	N2.2.1	N2.2.2	N2.3.1	N2.3.2	N2.3.3	N2.3.4
Unit 1 Consult with and advise clients									
Face shapes		X		X	X	X			X
Unit 2 Provide hair and scalp treatment services									
Analysis of constituents of products				X	X	X	X	X	X
Unit 5 Colour hair to create a variety of fashion looks									
Calculate proportions of peroxide to distilled water				X	X				
Unit 6 Style hair to create a variety of fashion looks									
Survey of clients and services provided over past month	X	X	X	X	X	X	X	X	X
Unit 7 Contribute to the effective running of the salon									
Survey	X	X	X			X	X	X	X

Communication

Activity	2.1a.1	2.1a.2	2.1a.3	2.1b.1	2.1b.2	2.1b.3	2.2.1	2.2.2	2.2.3	2.3.1	2.3.2	2.3.3	2.3.4
Unit 1 Consult with and advise clients													
Clients with problems!	X	X	X				X	X	X	X	X	X	X
Advising clients on suitable products				X	X	X				X	X	X	X
Group discussion on customer's rights	X	X	X										
Write a document on Consumer Protection Act										X	X	X	X
Lies and truths!	X	X	X										
Unit 2 Provide hair and scalp treatment services													
Group discussion on consultation with client	X	X	X										
Unit 3 Cut hair to create a variety of fashion looks													
Talk on health and safety in the salon				X	X	X				X	X	X	X
Unit 4 Perm hair to create a variety of fashion looks													
Talk to group on perming process				X	X	X							
Unit 5 Colour hair to create a variety of fashion looks													
Discussion on colouring faults	X	X	X										
Unit 6 Style hair to create a variety of fashion looks													
Advice on hair to a friend about to get married							X	X	X				
Unit 7 Contribute to the effective running of the salon													
Survey	X	X	X							X	X	X	X
Allocating work to junior colleagues	X	X	X							X	X	X	X

Activity	2.1a.1	2.1a.2	2.1a.3	2.1b.1	2.1b.2	2.1b.3	2.2.1	2.2.2	2.2.3	2.3.1	2.3.2	2.3.3	2.3.4
Unit 8 Contribute to maintaining health, safety and security of the salon environment													
Missing tips	X	X	X										
Employment rights and responsibilities													
Employment documents							X	X	X				
Equal opportunities							X	X	X				
Sickness and maternity payments							X	X	X				
Personnel records							X	X	X				
Health and safety							X	X	X				

SECTION 5: ADDITIONAL RESOURCES

Recommended websites

www.khake.com/page75.html – links to information on all theory units of hairdressing

www.keratin.com – information on hair and scalp disorders

www.beautyabout.com – professional hair products

www.hair-styles.org – hairstyle finder

wakcoll.ac.uk – face shape activities

www.city-&-guilds.org.uk – standards setting body for hairdressing qualifications

www.dti.gov.uk – Department of Trade and Industry

www.habia.org – the hairdressing and beauty industry authority; includes a range of information with links to other websites

www.bbc.co.uk/health – advice on avoiding skin diseases

www.lookfantastic.com – professional hairdressing products and advice

www.laurandp.co.uk – educational publications for development of professional hairdressing

www.vtct.org.uk – Vocational Training Charitable Trust; awarding body for professional hairdressing qualifications

www.fellowshiphair.com – 'who's who?' in hairdressing

www.hse.gov.uk – Health & Safety Executive

Useful books

S/NVQ Level 2 *Hairdressing with barbering* by Leah Palmer and Nicci Moorman (Heinemann, 2003)

S/NVQ Level 3 *Hairdressing, with barbering* by Gilly Ford and Helen Stewart (Heinemann, 2003)

Suggested magazines

Hairdresser's Journal

Creative Head

Black Beauty and Hair

Estetica/Cutting Edge

Client consultation checklist

Unit no ....

Client's name ....   Student's name ....

Date ....   Record card? Yes /No ....

Select client face shape:

Oval ☐

Round ☐

Square ☐

Rectangular ☐

Heart-shaped ☐

Diamond-shaped ☐

Pear-shaped ☐

Contraindications:

Skin sensitivities ☐   Skin disorders ☐   Incompatible products ☐

History of previous allergic reactions to colouring products ☐

Medical advice or instruction ☐   Other known allergies ☐

Scalp condition:

Possible disorder/adverse condition ....Dry/Flaky/Normal/Oily

Hair texture	Coarse ☐ Medium ☐ Fine ☐
Hair type	African Caribbean ☐ Caucasian/European ☐ Asian/Oriental ☐
Hair length	Very long ☐ Long ☐ Medium ☐ Short ☐
Hair condition	Normal ☐ Greasy ☐ Dry ☐
Volume	Thick ☐ Medium ☐ Thin ☐
Movement	Straight ☐ Wavy ☐ Curly ☐
Hair growth patterns	Nape whorl ☐ Widow's peak ☐ Cowlick ☐ Double crown ☐

	Testing procedures	Time taken for cutting:
Perm	Elasticity/porosity	
Tint/colour	Incompatibility	
Highlights	Skin test	
Lowlights	Pre-perm test	
Relaxing	Strand test Test cutting	-------------------------

Current look	Long	Medium	Short	Very short	Desired look	Long	Medium	Short	Very short
Layered					Layered				
Graduated					Graduated				
One-length					One-length				
Club cut					Club cut				
Razored					Razored				
Texturised					Texturised				
With fringe					With fringe				
Without fringe					Without fringe				

Shampooing/conditioning service **Equipment used:**	Products used:	**Conditioning technique:** Surface ☐ Penetrating ☐ Treatment ☐	Time taken:
Drying and styling hair Tools used: (including heated appliances):	Products used:	**Drying techniques:** Roller setting ☐ Pin curling ☐ Finger waving ☐ Blow drying ☐ Finger drying ☐	Time taken:
Perming Virgin hair ☐ Chemically treated ☐	Reconstructant used?	Rod size Winding method Perm used Acid or alkaline? Processing time With heat	Time taken (winding):
Neutralising	Equipment used:	**Product used:** Method of application Development time	Time taken:
Colouring Temporary ☐ Semi ☐ Quasi ☐ Permanent ☐ Hi-lift tint ☐ Bleach ☐	Product used/shade no: **Peroxide strength:**	Full head ☐ Re-growth ☐ Partial ☐ Hi/light ☐ Low/light ☐ Natural depth % of white Target shade Method of application Development time	Time taken:

INDEX